Cancer Medicine in an Ayurvedic Perspective: A Critical Overview

Edited By

Vaishali Kuchewar

*Datta Meghe Institute of Higher Education and Research
(Deemed to be University), Wardha
Maharashtra, India*

Gaurav Rajendra Sawarkar

*Datta Meghe Institute of Higher Education and Research
(Deemed to be University), Wardha
Maharashtra, India*

Padam Prasad Simkhada

*Global Consortium for Public Health and Research
School of Human and Health Sciences
University of Huddersfield
Queensgate, Huddersfield, UK*

&

Mahalaqua Nazli Khatib

*Datta Meghe Institute of Higher Education and Research
(Deemed to be University), Wardha
Maharashtra, India*

Cancer Medicine in an Ayurvedic Perspective: A Critical Overview

Editors: Vaishali Kuchewar, Gaurav Rajendra Sawarkar, Padam Prasad Simkhada and Mahalaqua Nazli Khatib

ISBN (Online): 978-981-5123-85-2

ISBN (Print): 978-981-5123-86-9

ISBN (Paperback): 978-981-5123-87-6

First published in 2023.

need for a court order if at any point you breach any terms of this License Agreement. In no event will any delay or failure by Bentham Science Publishers in enforcing your compliance with this License Agreement constitute a waiver of any of its rights.

3. You acknowledge that you have read this License Agreement, and agree to be bound by its terms and conditions. To the extent that any other terms and conditions presented on any website of Bentham Science Publishers conflict with, or are inconsistent with, the terms and conditions set out in this License Agreement, you acknowledge that the terms and conditions set out in this License Agreement shall prevail.

Bentham Science Publishers Pte. Ltd.
80 Robinson Road #02-00
Singapore 068898
Singapore
Email: subscriptions@benthamscience.net

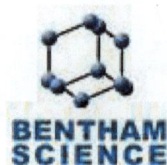

BENTHAM SCIENCE

CONTENTS

FOREWORD

The initiative and the effort are diligently expressed by the members of the faculty at the Mahatma Gandhi Ayurved College, Hospital and Research Centre, Sawangi Meghe, Wardha a constituent unit of Datta Meghe Institute of Higher Education and Research (Deemed University). Sawangi Meghe, Wardha is indeed not only laudable but also praiseworthy for the very cause it has been undertaken.

It is a matter of established common knowledge that there is an imperative need for the creation of a genuine and meaningful book titled **"Cancer Medicine in an Ayurvedic Perspective: A Critical Overview"** for the learners of Ayurvedic Sciences at various levels studying in various Ayurvedic Schools across the country. The content embodied in the book, which caters to the need of the learners, teachers and professionals in a free flowing manner is the core necessity as of now, which has remained unattended for reasons more than one.

The initiative undertaken by the teaching faculty of Mahatma Gandhi Ayurveda College, Hospital and Research Centre, needs to be viewed with, in the context of its relevance and consequence. To my understanding, the notable effort undertaken is timely, apt and also meaningful in its own way.

It is really a very benign and genuine effort on the part of all the contributing authors to compile all the relevant intellectual inputs on a significantly vital area and render them in such a free-flowing manner, so that it is easy to understand, decipher, grasp and assimilate by the learner, teacher, professionals and a casual reader, as well.

This has been singularly achieved by the authors by virtue of their writings which are in the handy textual format and are appropriately aligned so as to render the desired grasp and much sought-after understanding of the subject in an easy yet immaculate manner, which turns out to be the unique feature of the dedicated authorship, which makes it look and feel different from the other available reading material on the subject in vogue.

The authors have painfully brought all that was needed, relevant and vital pertaining to the thematic depiction of the subject at hand in a very deserving, appropriate, chronologically lucid manner. The chapterization vividly brings out the continuum in a logical and chronological manner. The entire team effort is embodied in single-minded devotion and un-paralleled dedication on their part, which speaks volumes about their intent to cater to the larger academic task and fill in the existing vacuum.

I am sure that this elegant piece of well-meaning and suitably documented scientific literature, appropriately illustrated by suitable diagrammatic and pictorial depictions wherever warranted embodied in the book format by the authors will make every user feel that he could avail himself all that he desired, needed and expected out of it.

I have no hesitation in putting on record my deep sense of appreciation for the effort undertaken by the authors in terms of a loud statement that they have evolved a satiety centre towards quenching the 'inquisitional thrust' in the domain of Ayurvedic Sciences as a whole in a genuinely exemplary and emulative manner.

Vedprakash Mishra
Pro-Chancellor
Datta Meghe Institute of Higher Education and Research (Deemed to be University)
Sawangi (Meghe), Wardha, Maharashtra, India

PREFACE

When a cancer patient comes to an Ayurveda practitioner with hope, they are often in a dilemma for its management. Many times, I searched books for the queries I had. In such a discussion, all had the same thought of writing a book on Cancer, which gives the basic information on Cancer from Ayurveda's perspective.

In the present world of increasing cancer prevalence, it is essential to have some alternative to prevent it and take care of the side effects of current treatment.

To help the practitioner and Ayurveda academician clear the Ayurveda concepts about Cancer, we came up with the book Cancer Medicine in an Ayurvedic Perspective: A Critical Overview. This book comprises nine chapters. It covered the Ayurveda perspective of understanding the etiopathogenesis of Cancer and its preventive and curative aspect. We sincerely hope that this book will help build confidence in the Ayurved fraternity to help cancer patients.

We would appreciate it if any discrepancy/deficiency which might have remained is brought to our notice. We also welcome suggestions for further improvement of the book.

Vaishali Kuchewar
Department of Kaychikitsa, Mahatma Gandhi Ayurved College
Hospital & Research Centre, Salod (H)
Datta Meghe Institute of Higher Education and Research (Deemed to be University)
Wardha, Maharashtra, India

Gaurav Rajendra Sawarkar
Department of Rachana Sharir Mahatma Gandhi
Ayurved College Hospital & Research Centre, Salod (H)
Datta Meghe Institute of Higher Education and Research (Deemed to be University)
Wardha, Maharashtra, India

Padam Prasad Simkhada
Global Consortium for Public Health and Research
School of Human and Health Sciences University of Huddersfield
Queensgate, Huddersfield, UK

&

Mahalaqua Nazli Khatib
Datta Meghe Institute of Higher Education and Research (Deemed to be University)
Wardha, Maharashtra, India

List of Contributors

Akshay Sudhir Pargaonkar
Department of Dravyaguna Vigyan, Mahatma Gandhi Ayurved College Hospital & Research Centre, Salod (H), Wardha, Maharashtra, 442001, India

Bharat Rathi
Department of Rasashastra & Bhaishajya Kalpana, Mahatma Gandhi Ayurved College Hospital & Research Centre, Salod (H), Wardha, Maharashtra, 442001, India

Bhagyashree R. Jibkate
Department of Rasashastra & Bhaishajya Kalpana, Mahatma Gandhi Ayurved College Hospital & Research Centre, Salod (H), Wardha, Maharashtra, 442001, India

Bhushan Mhaiskar
Department of Samhita and Siddhant, Mahatma Gandhi Ayurved College Hospital and Research Centre, Salod, Wardha, Maharashtra, India

Dhirajsingh S. Rajput
Central Council for Research in Ayurvedic Sciences (CCRAS), Ministry of AYUSH, New Delhi, India

Gaurav Rajendra Sawarkar
Department of Rachana Sharir, Mahatma Gandhi Ayurved College Hospital & Research Centre, Salod (H), Datta Meghe Institute of Higher Education and Research (Deemed to be University), Wardha, Maharashtra, India

Jagruti N.Chaple
Department of Kriya Sharir, Mahatma Gandhi Ayurved College, Hospital & Research Centre, Salod (H), Wardha, Maharashtra, India

Punam Sawarkar
Department of Panchakarma, Mahatma Gandhi Ayurved College, Hospital and Research Centre, Datta Meghe Institute of Higher Education and Research (Deemed to be University), Wardha, Maharashtra, India

Sadhana Misar Wajpeyi
Department of Kayachikitsa, Mahatma Gandhi Ayurved College Hospital and Research Centre, Salod (H), Wardha, Maharashtra, India

Sonali Chalakh
Department of Agadtantra, Mahatma Gandhi Ayurved College Hospital & Research Center, Wardha, Maharashtra, India

Seema H. Thakare
Department of Rognidan and Vikruti Vigyan, Mahatma Gandhi Ayurved College Hospital and Research Centre, Salod (H), Wardha, Maharashtra, India

Vaishali Kuchewar
Department of Kaychikitsa, Mahatma Gandhi Ayurved College, Hospital & Research Centre, Salod (H), Datta Meghe Institute of Higher Education and Research (Deemed to be University), Wardha, Maharashtra, India

CHAPTER 1

Cancer from Ayurveda Perspective

Bhushan Mhaiskar[1,*] and **Vaishali Kuchewar**[2]

[1] *Department of Samhita and Siddhant, Mahatma Gandhi Ayurved College Hospital and Research Centre, Salod, Wardha, Maharashtra, India*

[2] *Department of Kaychikitsa, Mahatma Gandhi Ayurved College, Hospital & Research Centre, Salod (H), Datta Meghe Institute of Higher Education and Research (Deemed to be University), Wardha, Maharashtra, India*

Abstract: Cancer is a leading cause of mortality among the world's population. Worldwide, 19.3 million new cancer cases and almost 10 million cancer deaths occurred in 2020. Cancer-like conditions are described in Ayurveda texts under the nomenclature of Arbuda and Asadhya Vrana (Non-healing ulcers). Mithya Ahara and Vihara vitiate Tridosha, responsible for different types of Arbuda. According to dhatu involvement, various types of Arbuda are defined. If Arbuda is left untreated, it is ultered into Asadhya Vrana. Acharya Sushruta has also advised multiple surgeries for Arbuda.

Keywords: Ayurveda, Arbuda, Asadhya vrana, Dosha.

INTRODUCTION

The term 'cancer' originated from the ancient Greek 'kapkivoc', which means 'crab' and 'tumor'. It includes various diseases involving abnormal cell growth with the capacity to spread to other parts of the body. Cancer can be correlated with the conditions described in Ayurvedic literature, such as Charak, Sushruta, *etc*. The diseases falling specifically under the category of cancer are Arbuda (lumps or swelling) and Asadhya Vrana (Non-healing ulcers) [1].

ARBUDA

According to Sushrut, it is a gradually increasing mass, spherical in shape, fixed with deeper structure, generally non-suppurative, occasionally painful, and can occur in any part of the body. It is caused due to vitiation of Tridosa and can involve Rakta and Mamsa Dhatu.

---

[*] **Corresponding author Bhushan Mhaiskar:** Department of Samhita and Siddhant, Mahatma Gandhi Ayurved College Hospital and Research Centre, Salod, Wardha, Maharashtra, India; E-mail: dr.bhu2050@gmail.com

Samprapti (etiopathogenesis) of Arbuda: Mithya Ahara and Vihara vitiate Tridosha involving various Dhatus (Rakta, Mamsa, Meda, *etc.*) result in different types of Arubuda. Though there is the involvement of Tridosha, Sushruta has mentioned the predominant involvement of Kapha Dosha, which is painless and non-suppurative.

Trauma has also been mentioned as another causative factor for the development of Mamsarbuda, such as Galaganda, Gandamala, Arbuda, Granthi, and Adhimamsa.

Classification of Arbuda

Arbuda can be classified according to:

1. Predominance of Dosha.

2. Involvement of Dhatu.

3. Site of Arbuda

4. Prognosis of Arbuda

According to the predominance of Dosha, there are four types of Arbuda. Vataja, Pittaja, Kaphaja, and Tridosaja are diagnosed based on symptomatology.

According to the involvement of Dhatu (tissue or cells): Arbuda is described as:

1. Medaja Arbuda (excess growth of fatty tissue).

2. Mamsaja Arbuda (excess growth of muscular tissue).

3. Raktarbuda (excess growth of blood cells).

Sushrut has mentioned various Arbuda as per the involvement of organs, such as Nasarbuda (Tumor of the nose), Karnarbuda (Tumor of the ear), Vartmarbuda (Tumor of the eyelid), Ostharbuda (Tumor of the lip), Galarbuda (Tumor of the throat), Mukharbuda (Tumor of buccal mucosa) and Sirarbuda (Tumors of head or brain). Arbuda of the genital organ has also been stated under "Shuka Dosha". It is caused due to the inappropriate use of various types of 'Linga vrddhikar Yoga'.

Based on the prognosis of the Arbuda, it is categorized as:

1. Sadhya (curable)

2. Asadhya (Incurable)

Mamsarbuda, Raktarbuda and Tridoshaj arbuda of any site are considered as Asadhya (incurable).

Sadhya Arbuda may develop into Asadhya Arbuda. It is described as "Adhyarbuda" or "Dvirarbuda". If Arbuda is formed near the primary growth, it is called Adhyarbuda, whereas Dvirarbuda is a similar type of growth at different places. It can be considered metastasis.

ASADHYA VRANA

It resembles malignant ulcers as per the similarity in clinical features. Susruta has described the nature of Asadhya Vrana being chronic and having characteristics of raised edges and various types of discharge. Sometimes, other features are also present, such as painful respiration, anorexia, chronic cough, and cachexia, which suggest cancer metastasis [2].

The following diseases are also called Asadhya. Its manifestation is also similar to a malignancy.

1. Mamsaja Ostha is a thick bulging mass that may convert into lip ulcers. It can be considered lip cancer.

2. Alasa: It is deep-seated swelling of the tongue caused due to vitiation of Rakta and Kapha. It has a fishy odor discharge and destroys the surrounding structures. It resembles epidermoid tumors of salivary glands.

3. Mamsa Kacchapa: It is a big, painful palate swelling due to incurable vitiation of Kapha. It can compare with a tumor of the hard palate.

4. Galaudha: It is an extensive swelling in the throat due to the vitiation of Rakta and Kapha. It becomes fatal due to difficulty in swallowing and respiration. It can be correlated with malignant growth at the oropharynx.

5. Lingarsa is a growth of fleshy mass with blood discharge on the external genitalia. It closely resembles a papillary carcinoma.

6. Asadhya Pradara – It can be correlated with carcinoma of the uterus because of its clinical features of excessive vaginal discharge of various colors, consistency and odor, and associated emaciation.

Treatment Principle

According to Ayurveda, no disease can manifest without an imbalance of Tridosha. It is necessary to specify the involvement of type of Dosha, Dhatu,

Strotas, and Agni to plan the treatment accordingly. With the medicinal treatment, Sushrut has also advised various surgeries wherever necessary [3].

CONCLUSION

In Ayurved literature, various conditions like Arbuda and Asadhya Vrana are documented, similar to Cancer. Mithya ahar and vihar (imbalanced diet and lifestyle) are the basic etiological factors. These factors are responsible for the vitiation of dosha, leading to the involvement of various Strotas and Dhatu. The nomenclature of Arbud depends on the involvement of Dhatu. Depending on the type of Arbud, various treatment options (including surgery) are mentioned.

REFERENCES

[1]   Online Etymology Dictionary. Available from: www.etymonline.com

[2]   Shastri KA. Samhita S. Sharir sthana, 3rd chapter, Chaukhambha Sanskrit sansthan Varansi, Reprint 2010; 27.

[3]   Srikantha Murthy KR. Chaukhambha Krishnadas Ashtanga hridayam, Vol. III, Uttara Sthana, Granthi Arbuda Sleepada Apachi Nadi Vijnaniya. Reprint 2014; 29(15): 274-80.

CHAPTER 2

Overview of Cancer

Vaishali Kuchewar[1,*]

[1] Department of Kaychikitsa, Mahatma Gandhi Ayurved College, Hospital & Research Centre, Salod (H), Datta Meghe Institute of Higher Education and Research (Deemed to be University), Wardha, Maharashtra, India

Abstract: The characteristics of cancer cells are continuous cell growth due to their non-responding nature to the signals of stopping the growth or apoptosis, the ability to spread in other parts of the body, and immortality of cells because of their capacity to restore their telomeres. The clinical features depend on the size and location of cancer and the presence or absence of metastasis. Local and systemic symptoms rely on the tumor mass and the body's response to cancer, respectively. Cancer is classified according to the tissue involved, like Carcinomas, Sarcomas, Myeloma, Leukemia, Lymphoma, Germ cell tumor, and blastoma. The globally recognized standard to classify the extent of cancer spread is called T.N.M. Classification. It applies to many solid tumor cancers but is not relevant to leukemia and the central nervous systems tumor. The tumor can be diagnosed with tests like mammograms, Pap smears, Tumor markers, Bone scans, MRI, Tissue biopsies, and PET-CT scans. The treatment depends on the type and stage of cancer and the patient's overall health. Common treatment modalities are surgery, radiation, and chemotherapy. Other treatments are targeted/biological therapies, hematopoietic stem cell transplants, angiogenesis inhibitors, cryosurgery, and photodynamic therapy. Every treatment has its risks, benefits, and side effects.

Keywords: Blastoma, Cancer, Chemotherapy, Germ cell tumor, Leukemia, Lymphoma, Metastasis, Myeloma, Radiation, Sarcomas, Surgery, TNM classification.

INTRODUCTION

Cancer is the uncontrolled growth of abnormal cells in the body. It often forms a mass or a lump called a neoplasm or tumor. Every mass or lump is not cancerous. The non-cancerous lump is called benign. It is restricted and risky if it compresses vital organs like the brain. Malignant neoplasms are commonly called cancer. They invade and destroy the surrounding tissue. Cancer cells spread to other sites

---

* **Corresponding author Vaishali Kuchewar**: Department of Kaychikitsa, Mahatma Gandhi Ayurved College, Hospital & Research Centre, Salod (H), Datta Meghe Institute of Higher Education and Research (Deemed to be University), Wardha, Maharashtra, India; E-mail: vkuchewar@gmail.com

through the lymphatic system and the bloodstream. And, if left untreated or become unresponsive to treatment, they will generally prove to be fatal.

Following are the characteristics of cancer cells:

1. The continuous growth of cells due to their non-responding nature to the signals of stopping the growth or apoptosis.

2. Ability to occupy nearby tissue.

3. Ability to spread to other parts of the body.

4. Immortality of cells because of their capacity to restore their telomeres.

Causes

Genetic mutations cause 95% of cancers due to environmental and lifestyle factors. The other is due to inherited genetics [1].

Risk Factors

- Exposure to cancer-causing chemicals and radiation
- Excessive sun exposure
- Certain types of diet & physical inactivity
- Smoking
- Certain viruses like human papillomavirus (HPV)

Clinical Features

The clinical features depend on the size and location of cancer and the presence or absence of metastasis. Local and systemic symptoms depend on the tumor's mass and the body's response to cancer, respectively.

Standard clinical features are:

- Fatigue
- Pain
- Fever
- Unintentional weight loss or weight gain
- Lumps or tumors
- Difficulty in swallowing
- Changes in bowel or bladder function
- Persistent hoarseness or cough
- Unexplained bleeding or discharge

CATEGORIES OF CANCER

Cancer is further classified according to the tissue involved [2].

1. Carcinomas

2. Sarcomas

3. Myeloma

4. Leukemia

5. Lymphoma

6. Germ cell tumor

7. Blastoma

Carcinoma

Occurs in epithelial tissues. 80% to 90% of cancers are of this category. It includes cancer of the prostate, lung, colon, skin, breast, and most common skin cancers, *i.e.*, basal cell carcinoma and squamous cell carcinoma.

Sarcoma

Occurs in connective tissues like fat, blood vessels, bones, cartilage, and muscles. Osteosarcoma, Ewing sarcoma, Kaposi sarcoma, Rhabdomyosarcoma, and leiomyosarcoma are some examples.

Myeloma

It occurs in plasma cells in the bone marrow. In this condition, plasma cells grow out of control in the bone marrow damaging it and can destroy the bone.

Leukemia

It is also called blood cancer. Numerous abnormal blood cells are found in the bloodstream.

Lymphoma

It is related to the cells of the immune system. It includes Hodgkin lymphoma and non-Hodgkin lymphoma.

Germ Cell Tumor

It is a cancer of pluripotent cells; it is commonly found in the ovary called dysgerminoma or in a testicle known as seminoma.

Blastoma

It is a tumor of primitive, incompletely differentiated (or precursor) cells. It is more common in children. Some examples of blastoma are hepatoblastoma, medulloblastoma, nephroblastoma, and neuroblastoma.

STAGES OF CANCER

The globally recognized standard to classify the extent of cancer spread is called TNM Classification. It applies to many solid tumor cancers but is not relevant to leukemia and the central nervous system's tumor.

TNM has the following alphanumeric codes:

- T (Tumor): Size of the original (primary) tumor and its invasion of nearby tissues.
- N (lymph nodes): Involvement of regional lymph nodes.
- M (Metastasis): Spreading of cancer from one site to another of the body.

The TNM classification is correlated to one of the following five stages:

- Stage 0: It refers to cancer "*in situ*", It means restricted to the site of origin and does not invade other tissues.
- Stage I to Stage III includes larger tumors or a greater extent of disease. Cancer may spread to the regional lymph nodes or organs in these stages.
- Stage IV: In this stage, the cancer is spread to lymph nodes or organs far away from the site of origin.

DIAGNOSIS OF CANCER

Following are some tests used to diagnose various types of cancer:

- **Mammogram:** It is a specific type of breast imaging to detect and diagnose breast cancer in women.
- **Pap smear Test:** It is a screening procedure for uterine cervical cancer. A sample of cells from the cervix is taken to check the abnormalities indicative of cervical cancer.

- **Tumor Marker Test:** Tumor markers are specific proteins found in higher levels in the blood, urine, or tissues of people with cancer. These are also called biomarkers.
- **Bone Scan:** This test includes a small amount of a radioactive substance injected into a vein. It identifies the suspected cancer area where too much or too little radioactive substance has been absorbed.
- **MRI:** It is an imaging test. It produces computer-generated pictures of the body to discover and measure the tumor size.
- **Tissue Biopsy:** It is a procedure to remove a piece of tissue to analyze cancer diagnosis.
- **PET-CT Scan:** It is an imaging test useful for detecting cancer. Cancer cells show bright spots on PET scans because of this high level of chemical activity.

TREATMENT

The treatment depends on the type and stage of cancer and the patient's overall health [3].

The common treatment modalities are:

- Surgery
- Radiation and
- Chemotherapy.

Other treatments include:

- Targeted/biological therapies,
- Hematopoietic stem cell transplants,
- Angiogenesis inhibitors,
- Cryosurgery, and
- Photodynamic therapy.

Every treatment has its risks, benefits, and side effects.

Surgery

It is commonly performed to remove the tumor, determine the exact size of cancer, and invade nearby structures or lymph nodes. Surgery is often combined with chemotherapy and radiation. Debulking surgery is advised for the tumor near the vital organ. Similarly, palliative surgery is performed in advanced cancer cases to reduce the discomfort of a cancerous tumor. Debulking and palliative surgeries are not curative; they only minimize the effects of cancer.

Radiation

It is ionizing radiation therapy to kill malignant cells. Radiation can be delivered externally or internally. Internal radiation can be given by placing radioactive material inside the body near cancer cells (brachytherapy) or by administering radioactive medication by mouth or intravenously. The radioactive material travels directly to the cancerous tissue. Radioactive iodine (I-131 for thyroid cancer) and strontium-89 (for bone cancer) are examples.

Radiation therapy can control cell growth. It damages the DNA of cancerous tissue resulting in cellular death. The response of radiation depends on its radiosensitivity. Highly radiosensitive cancer cells are killed very fast by radiation. Some types of cancer are markedly radio-resistant, so higher doses of radiation are required.

Side Effects

Radiation is a painless therapy. Its low dose has minimal or no side effects. Higher doses can cause acute or long-term side effects.

Acute Side Effects

1. Nausea and vomiting are related to the treatment of abdominal cancer or radiation to head and neck tumors as these are nausea-producing structures.

2. Damage to the epithelial surfaces - Radiation therapy may damage epithelial surfaces of the skin, oral mucosa, pharyngeal, bowel mucosa, and ureter.

3. Infertility - The gonads (ovaries and testicles) are very sensitive to radiation. They may be unable to produce gametes due to the direct radiation exposure.

Late Side Effects

Radiation damages blood vessels and connective tissue, causing the following.

1. Fibrosis – The elasticity of irradiated tissues is decreased, causing the process of fibrosis.

2. Epilation (hair loss) results in radiation doses above 1 Gy.

3. Dryness - The common side effects are dry mouth (xerostomia), dry eyes (xerophthalmia), and dryness in the vaginal mucosa. It severely affects a patient's quality of life.

4. Lymphedema is the most common complication of radiation therapy in breast cancer.

5. Cardiovascular disease – Radiation may cause myocardial fibrosis, coronary and peripheral artery disease, and valvular disease.

6. Cognitive decline is found in head radiation therapy in children from 5 to 11 years of age group.

7. Radiation enteropathy – Radiation causes fibrosis and vascular changes in the intestine producing diarrhea, malabsorption, and steatorrhea.

8. Radiation-induced polyneuropathy - In the initial phase, there is nerve demyelination due to microvascular injury. In the next step, nerve compression occurs due to uncontrolled fibrous growth.

9. Radiation necrosis – Direct or indirect damage of blood vessels due to radiation causes infarction to result in necrosis.

Chemotherapy

It refers to the different medications used to treat cancer. It aims to slow cancer growth, prevent it from spreading, and relieve cancer-associated symptoms such as pain.

In chemotherapy, the medications can be given by mouth, intravenously (IV), or topically. Sometimes chemotherapy is delivered regionally, directly to the area that needs treatment, like intra-vesical therapy in bladder cancer.

Chemotherapy is usually administered in cycles for days, weeks, or months, with rest periods.

Following are the types of chemotherapy:

- Induction chemotherapy is the first-line cancer treatment with a chemotherapeutic drug. This type of chemotherapy is used for curative purposes.
- Combined modality chemotherapy: It is advised with surgery or other therapies.
- Consolidation chemotherapy is given for the patient's recovery, and the same remission drug is continued.
- Intensification chemotherapy is similar to consolidation chemotherapy, but a different drug is used.
- Combination chemotherapy: It includes different drugs simultaneously. The advantage of this therapy is to minimize drug resistance. Also, drug toxicity can

be reduced by using a low dose of each medicine.

- Neo-adjuvant chemotherapy is local chemotherapy given before surgery to shrink the primary tumor.
- Adjuvant chemotherapy: It is local chemotherapy given after surgery or radiotherapy. It is used explicitly in the cases of risk of recurrence.
- Maintenance chemotherapy: It is a repeated low-dose treatment to prolong remission.
- Salvage chemotherapy (palliative chemotherapy) is not given for a curative purpose but to decrease tumor load and increase life expectancy.

Adverse Effects

1. Immunosuppression and myelosuppression: Most chemotherapeutic regimens cause depression in the immune system by suppressing the bone marrow. Sometimes, chemotherapy is postponed due to a significantly low level of the immune system.

2. Neutropenic enterocolitis (typhlitis) is a life-threatening intestinal infection caused due to the suppression of the immune system. Its clinical features include nausea, vomiting, diarrhea, fever, chills, or abdominal pain. It is often fatal if not treated early.

3. Anemia is caused due to chemotherapy having side effects of myelosuppression, bleeding tendency, or hemolysis.

4. Hair loss (alopecia): It is a temporary effect. After a few weeks of last treatment, hair usually starts to regrow; but there may be alteration in color. Sometimes hair may be curly, known as "chemo curls."

5. Infertility: Some types of chemotherapy cause infertility in females.

6. Teratogenicity: Chemotherapy causes teratogenic during the first trimester of pregnancy. Second- and third-trimester exposure does not usually increase the teratogenic risk, but it may increase the risk of various complications of pregnancy and fetal myelosuppression. In males, no genetic defects or congenital malformations are found in their children who conceived after therapy.

7. Peripheral neuropathy: 30 and 40% of people experience chemotherapy-induced peripheral neuropathy (CIPN). The patient may experience pain, tingling sensation, and cold sensitivity. The severity of it depends on the type of drug and its duration of use.

8. Tumor lysis syndrome is a rapid breakdown of cancer cells that excessively release chemicals like uric acid and potassium. It may lead to death if not diagnosed and treated early.

Other side effects include erythema, dry skin, dry mouth (xerostomia), water retention, and impotence.

Limitations

Chemotherapy does not always work. The blood-brain barrier obstructs the delivery of chemotherapy to the brain to protect it from harmful chemicals. Drug transporters pump out chemotherapy drugs, which reduces their efficacy in brain tumors. As cancer grows, the newly formed tumor vasculature is not proper, so it does not deliver the drug in the required quantity.

OTHER TREATMENT THERAPIES

In addition to surgery, radiation, and chemotherapy, other therapies are used to treat cancer. These include:

Targeted or Biological Therapies

It boosts the body's immune system while minimizing damage to normal, healthy cells. Monoclonal antibodies, immune-modulating drugs, vaccines, and cytokines are examples of targeted or biological therapies.

Targeted therapy blocks the growth of cancer cells by interfering with specific targeted molecules needed for carcinogenesis and tumor growth rather than by only interfering with all rapidly dividing cells (*e.g.*, with traditional chemotherapy). Because most agents for targeted therapy are biopharmaceuticals, the term biologic therapy is sometimes synonymous with targeted therapy when used in the context of cancer therapy.

Another form of targeted therapy involves using nano-engineered enzymes to bind to a tumor cell such that the body's natural cell degradation process can digest the cell, virtually eliminating it from the body.

Targeted cancer therapies are expected to be more effective than older forms of treatments and less harmful to normal cells.

There are targeted therapies for lung cancer, colorectal cancer, head and neck cancer, breast cancer, multiple myeloma, lymphoma, prostate cancer, melanoma, and other cancers.

Hematopoietic Stem Cell Transplants

It involves the infusion of stem cells into a cancer patient after the bone marrow has been destroyed by high-dose chemo and radiation.

HSC transplants are used to treat cancers and other immune system disorders.

Hematopoietic stem cells are found in the bone marrow of adults, especially in the pelvis, femur, and sternum. They are also found in umbilical cord blood and, in small numbers, in peripheral blood.

Stem and progenitor cells can be taken from the pelvis at the iliac crest using a needle and syringe. The cells can be removed as a liquid, or they can be removed *via* a core biopsy. Hematopoietic stem cells are essential to hematopoiesis. They can replenish all blood cell types.

Angiogenesis Inhibitors

These medications slow the growth of new blood vessels that cancerous tumors need to grow.

Cryosurgery

Extreme cold is applied to kill precancerous and cancerous cells.

Photodynamic Therapy

It is the application of laser energy of a specific wavelength to tissue that has been treated with a photosensitizing agent. This medication makes cancerous tissue susceptible to destruction with laser treatment. Photodynamic therapy selectively destroys cancer cells while minimizing the damage to normal, healthy tissues nearby.

CANCER PREVENTION

It is defined as active measures to decrease cancer risk. The majority of cancer is due to environmental risk factors. Many of these environmental factors are controllable lifestyle choices. Thus, cancer is generally preventable. Greater than 30% of cancer deaths could be prevented by avoiding risk factors, including tobacco, excess weight/obesity, poor diet, physical inactivity, alcohol, sexually transmitted infections, and air pollution. Some environmental causes are uncontrollable, such as naturally occurring background radiation and cancers caused through hereditary genetic disorders, and thus are not preventable with personal behavior.

CONCLUSION

Cancer cells can spread to other parts of the body, proliferate continuously, and restore their telomeres, making them immortal. The tumour and body cause local and systemic symptoms. Cancers include carcinomas, sarcomas, myelomas, leukaemia, lymphomas, germ cell tumours, and blastomas. T.N.M. Classification is the global cancer spread standard. Leukemia and central nervous system tumours are excluded. Mammograms, Pap smears, tumor markers, bone scans, MRIs, tissue biopsies, and PET-CT scans can detect tumors. Treatments include surgery, radiation, and chemotherapy. Hematopoietic stem cell transplants, angiogenesis inhibitors, cryosurgery, and photodynamic therapy are other options. Each treatment has pros and cons.

REFERENCES

[1]   Danaei G, Vander Hoorn S, Lopez AD, Murray CJ, Ezzati M. Causes of cancer in the world: comparative risk assessment of nine behavioral and environmental risk factors. Lancet 2005; 366(9499): 1784-93.
[http://dx.doi.org/10.7759/cureus.28875] [PMID: 36225498]

[2]   Wu S, Powers S, Zhu W, Hannun YA. Substantial contribution of extrinsic risk factors to cancer development. Nature 2016; 529(7584): 43-7.
[http://dx.doi.org/10.1038/nature16166]

[3]   Anand P, Kunnumakkara AB, Sundaram C, *et al.* Cancer is a preventable disease that requires major lifestyle changes. Pharm Res 2008; 25(9): 2097-116.
[http://dx.doi.org/10.1007/s11095-008-9661-9] [PMID: 18626751]

CHAPTER 3

The Concept of Epigenetics in Cancer

Gaurav Rajendra Sawarkar[1,*] and **Punam Sawarkar**[2]

[1] *Department of Rachana Sharir, Mahatma Gandhi Ayurved College Hospital & Research Centre, Salod (H), Datta Meghe Institute of Higher Education and Research (Deemed to be University), Wardha, Maharashtra, India*

[2] *Department of Panchakarma, Mahatama Gandhi Ayurved College, Hospital and Research Centre, Datta Meghe Institute of Higher Education and Research (Deemed to be University), Wardha, Maharashtra, India*

Abstract: Epigenetics is the term that comes before genetics. DNA is not able to determine the characteristics of a human being. The genotype corresponds to Prakriti by birth, and the phenotype corresponds to the psychophysiological constitution of Prakrit. The features and properties of RNA represent the Tridosha at the cellular level, which can be identified under the heading of mRNA, tRNA, and protein. There are four significant factors, *i.e.*, lifestyle and behavior, diet and digestion, stress, and environmental factors responsible for changes in the phenotype that led to changes in the genotypic expressions without changing the basic structure of DNA.

Nowadays, changing lifestyles, food habits, stress factors, uncontrolled pesticides used in the agricultural field, global warming, and undue environmental changes lead to epigenetic changes in humans. Ayurveda addresses solutions to the affecting factors by adopting the basic principles of Ayurveda, including daily routine, behavior, diet plan, exercise, meditation, medications, purification therapies, *etc.* The integration of the Indian system and the current medical system facilitates optimum health and stability for humanity. Further research on modalities, drugs, formulations, and herbs explained in Ayurveda for affective gene expression is needed to fulfill various cancers' desired management.

Keyword: Ayurveda, Cancer, Epigenetic, Prakriti.

INTRODUCTION

Epigenetics is the term that comes before genetics, which can regulate the organism preceding genetics. DNA is not able to determine the characteristics of a human being. Because the factors like environment, stress issues, nutrition, medicine, and many other surrounding stimuli influence organisms' responses like

---

* **Corresponding author Gaurav Rajendra Sawarkar:** Department of Rachana Sharir, Mahatma Gandhi Ayurved College Hospital & Research Centre, Salod (H), Datta Meghe Institute of Higher Education and Research (Deemed to be University), Wardha, Maharashtra, India; E-mail: drsawarkar.gaurav@gmail.com

DNA, we can say that nature and nurture are equally important in humans' observed responses. Accordingly, humans are affected by both epigenetics and genetic factors. Various researchers observed that some diseases' causative factors are epigenetic influences like lifestyle, diet, habits, and addictions [1]. This means genetic factors are not the final repository responsible for the health status of human beings. In today's era, most diseases labeled as lifestyle disorders, which indicate faulty lifestyles, give rise to many problems. If the host body has a favorable environment, such types of conditions transpire in the body. More than ninety percent of diseases like cancer, cardiovascular, and diabetes are the consequences of a faulty lifestyle and not merely because of inheritance. Hence, it can be concluded that epigenetic factors could override genetic factors.

CONCEPT OF EPIGENETICS

In modern science, it is considered that epigenetic alterations or mechanisms have regulated gene expressions. These alterations include genomic DNA, methylation, and post-translational modification of histone tails, which should be within higher-order chromatin and non-coding RNAs that regulate the gene expressions. Disturbed epigenetic mechanism causes various human pathologies, but their role in mitochondrial pathogenesis is still undefined. The epigenome in the mitochondrial disease pathology is essential to the affected epigenetic mechanism. Some cancer research studies conclude that mitochondrial defects are associated with epigenetic alteration within the nuclear genome, which plays a confounding complex role linked with mitochondrial diseases [2].

Most of the activities in the body are controlled by epigenetics, which drives the changes in gene expression. Prakriti is the Ayurved psychophysiological constitution in the form of a phenotype related to DNA. 'Karma', *i.e.*, action, involves the process of epigenetics, represents Newton's Third Law of Motion: For every step, there is an equal and opposite reaction and also the idiom "As you sow, so shall you reap" for the epigenetics changes in DNA expressions and its transmutability in future progeny. The life-affecting factors like lifestyle and behavior, diet and digestion, stress, and environmental factors disturbed the gene expressions. If human beings control their actions positively, which keeps body physiology in harmony, it means in a balanced state and preventing Vikruti, *i.e.*, disease manifestation. The imbalance state affects both the phenotype and the expression of the genotype; by controlling the above-mentioned affecting factor, one can reverse unwanted changes in the genetic expression. Each individual has the responsibility of their health to follow the guidelines mentioned in the prevention system of Ayurveda regarding individual Prakriti, which can protect undesirable changes in the phenotype and gene expression [3].

Epigenetics in Cancer

DNA is the chromatin structure in the form of genetic information organized in the cell. This organization significantly influences the abilities of the genes regarding their activation or silence form. Recent studies regarding epigenetics conclude that human cancer cells shelter epigenetic abnormalities and many genetic alterations, interact in all stages of cancer, and encourage cancer progression. Decades ago, cancer was considered a gene origin, but current research suggests that epigenetic alterations may be the initiating factor in some cancers. Many scholars are taking the initiative to recognize the concept of epigenetics and its role in cancer progression [4, 5].

Epigenetics and Phenotype

Epigenetics studies transmissible alterations in gene expression (means activation and inactivation of genes) that do not change the DNA sequence. Still, they are accountable for phenotype changes without a change in the genotype, which is entirely responsible for affected genes read by the cells. Phenotype is the individual's characteristics like height, eye color, blood type, etc. The genetic contribution to the expression of the phenotype is known as the genotype. The determination of characteristics is done based on genotype and environmental factors. Epigenetics explores the dynamic association between the environment and gene expression. The gene expressions are controlled at the chromosome level, which means which part of the DNA is allowed to read (transcription) to produce proteins (translation). As a result, genes may turn on or off because of the external modification of DNA. These modifications cannot change the DNA sequence but can control the expressions of the genes. Epigenetic changes are the outcome of DNA methylation and interaction between DNA and protein, *i.e.*, Histone. In short, DNA methylation is nothing but the epigenetic alteration that is linked with the process of histone modification, chromatin structure, and RNA interference. All these processes regulate gene transcription from embryonic to the consequent development of the body [6].

The Underlying Philosophy of Epigenetics

Ancient science, Ayurveda, and Vedic knowledge offer a philosophical understanding of the creation, sequence, and alteration of the universe and the urges of nature. The human being consists of two basic features: never changing and ever-changing things. The body's physique and inner perception constantly alter things; however, the deep inner consciousness is entirely constant and not alterable. DNA is the silent core part like Prakriti, which can express genes. DNA is the genetic code with all information of an individual, and its expression is a part of its knowledge. In the process of expression, two strands of DNA divide to form messenger RNA, *i.e.*, the transcription process, and then transfer RNA enables the translation process to create amino acids that unite to form proteins. DNA does not do anything, or nothing changes the structure and makes the expression part, *i.e.*, phenotype. The external factors influence DNA expressions because of the impact of epigenetics, the changes in lifestyle, diet, digestion, tobacco smoking, alcohol consumption, environmental pollutants, psychological stress, working in the night shift, mental stress, etc. The Prakriti is a unique entity with different characteristics per Dosha's predominant characteristics. The external environment, unwholesome food, and faulty lifestyle vitiate the Dosha and create disease conditions; these are all expressions associated with specific Prakriti [6, 7].

OVERVIEW OF PERSONALIZED MEDICINE

Ayurveda has specialized treatment for every disease individually, as every person has their own identity with a different constitution. The constitution of the body, Prakrit, is based on the predominance of Tridosha. It provides specific classified phenotypes collectively considered as genotypes. Similarly, the drugs are also classified according to their Rasa (taste), Guna (property), Virya (potency), Vipaka (post-digestive form), and Prabhava (effect other than that of prescribed properties).

Considering the Prakriti of individuals, the properties and action of drugs, the treatment can be planned in Ayurveda. Unlike modern treatment having various responses, the same drug should be designed for the same disease. This personalized medicine concept is only explained in ancient science, effectively filling the gap between inter-individual variations and drug response. It needs time to intervene in the experiential knowledge of scholars in personalized medicine for the proficiency and well-being of society. Aside from genetic inherited variations, the drug response is influenced by alteration in genes' function without changing the DNA sequence. These alterations result from RNA inactivation, histone modification, and DNA methylation. Therefore, most researchers are kin to map the DNA methylation pattern in different diseases to mark the epigenetic indicators of most common conditions and drug response patterns and streamline the way towards personalized medicine. Epigenomics therapy has much potential to treat patients with personalized treatment and broader access to screening and prevention strategies in the more general population.

Pharmacogenetics is the study related to the pharmacokinetics and pharmacodynamics of DNA sequences in inter-individual variations. Some studies conclude that the genetic variation in drug targets may reflect the drug's efficiency by revealing polymorphic variations in genes that encode transporters' functions, metabolizing enzymes, receptors, and other proteins. Drug discovery, therapeutic response, and pharmacological processes can be studied with genomic technologies, known as pharmacogenomics. It is the basis of personalized medicine and its utility at the individual level. On the other hand, Ayurgenomics is the newer term conceptualized under the integration of genomics and Ayurveda principles. There are some challenges to Ayurgenomics, similar to the establishment of a correlation between DNA and Prakriti, enzymes involved in the metabolism of drugs genotypes and Prakriti, so advance research studies should be planned on such topics to clarify fundamental differences and the similarities between pharmacogenomics and Ayurgenomics to carry out personalized treatment pattern virtually worldwide [7].

Prakriti-based and personalized medicine are both essential for health promotion and disease prevention. Epigenomics facilitates the study of the role of genes, proteins, metabolic pathways, and their variations responsible for disease conditions and finding out non-genetic factors involved in human physiology. In the Ayurveda context, Ayurgenomics is explained very well, considering its usability, delivery time, targeted organ or system, and Prakriti of the patient. With this concept, one can change the global health wisdom by offering diet habits, lifestyle modifications, and medicine as per the type of individual Prakriti [6].

BIOACTIVE DIETARY COMPONENTS AND EPIGENETIC TARGETS

Some researches show the chemopreventive and anticancer properties of beverages, fruits, vegetables, and other diet components. The variety of nutrients plays a vital role in regulating normal and pathologic processes in the body and preventing and treating various cancers [8]. The summarized part of some common bioactive dietary agents and their epigenetic targets on various cancers is mentioned in Table **1**.

Table 1. List of dietary agents and their epigenetic effect.

SN	Dietary Agent	Epigenetic Effect on Cancer
1	Parsley	DNMT inhibitor
2	Garlic	HDAC inhibitor
3	Turmeric	DNMT inhibitor, HDAC, and HAT inhibitor
4	Green tea (Camellia Sinensis)	DNMT inhibitor, HAT activator
5	Soybean	DNMT inhibitor, HDAC inhibitor, and HAT activator
6	Tomatoes	Demethylates the GSTP1, RARβ2, and HIN-1 genes in breast cancer cells

(Table 1) cont.....

SN	Dietary Agent	Epigenetic Effect on Cancer
7	Red/Black grapes	DNMT inhibitor, SIRT1 activator
8	Milk thistle	SIRT1 activator
9	Cruciferous vegetables like Brussels sprouts, cabbage, cauliflower, radish, turnips	DNMT inhibitor, HDAC inhibitor

*DNMT-DNA methyltransferases, HDAC - histone deacetylase, HAT - Histone acetylase, GSTP1 - Glutathione-S-transferase pi, RARβ - Retinoic acid receptor β, SIRT1 - Sirtuin 1

Besides these bioactive components, many common fruits and vegetables also have an epigenetic effect on cancer through DNMT inhibitors or histone modification.

Moreover, new treatment modalities like immunotherapy enhanced the ERV demethylation effect by having Vitamin C as a co-factor. As per observation, 60% of cancer patients have a vitamin C deficiency. It also suggests that dietary supplements help in overcoming vitamin C deficiency and act as epigenetic therapy in many patients.

EPIGENETIC THERAPY FOR CANCER

In cancer, various epigenetic changes were found, which are reversible. With the help of epigenetic therapy, there will be the possibility of treatment aiming to reverse the epigenetic aberrations in the body. Many drugs have recently been discovered for epigenetic medicine to restore the normal epigenome, stopover, and reverse DNA methylation and histone modification. DNA methylation inhibitors, with cytotoxic agents 5-azacytidine (5-aza-CR) and 5-aza-2'-deoxycytidine (5-aza-CdR), induce gene expression for the treatment of cancer. Present epigenetic drugs showed weak inhibitory potential, which indicates a need to discover a new potent drug in epigenetic therapy. For this purpose, various HDAC inhibitors like depsipeptide and phenylbutyrate are overcoming the shortcoming of the treatment. The combination treatment, DNA methylation, and HDAC inhibitors have been more effective than different uses. HMT inhibitor, another well-versed therapy, was selectively target the cancer cell treatment. miRNA can regulate aberrant epigenetic changes and restore normal epigenomes in the body. Though there is a significant issue regarding the efficient delivery methods, efficient vehicle molecules are required for the targeted delivery of synthetic miRNA [9].

According to Ayurveda, meditation provides physical, mental, and spiritual well-being and activates the inner consciousness, which connects with the deep inner self. The meditation facilitates the epigenetic feedback loop in the body cell, deep to the inner self, *i.e.*, DNA offers inner peace and bliss, which eliminates collective stress, surpasses senses, intellect, and ego, and reaches the pure consciousness [6].

Ayurveda also promotes herbs and spices; recent research shows medicinal and value-aided epigenetic properties. Ginger has neuroprotective, neurotrophic, and anti-inflammatory properties containing bioactive components regulating histone H3 acetylation, suppressing histone deacetylase expressions HDAC1and increasing the expression of HSP70, which improve neurological activities. Other dietary ingredients like honey, saffron, and ghee regulate epigenetic factors. Extensive research studies are required to find dietary chemopreventive drugs and other preventive tools mentioned in Ayurveda, which can bridge the gap between treatments and reduce discomfort, imbalance, and adverse effects [10].

CONCLUSION

It is concluded that the genotype and phenotype correspond to the Prakriti by birth and the psychophysiological constitution of Prakrit, respectively. The features and properties of RNA (mRNA, tRNA, and protein) represent the Tridosha at the cellular level. There are four significant factors, lifestyle and behavior, diet and digestion, stress, and environmental factors responsible for changes in the phenotype that led to changes in the genotypic expressions without changing the basic structure of DNA. Ayurveda addresses solutions to the affecting factors by adopting the basic principles of Ayurveda. The integration of the Indian system and the current medical system facilitates optimum health and stability for humanity. Further research on modalities, drugs, formulations, and herbs explained in Ayurveda for affective gene expression is needed to fulfill various cancers' desired management.

REFERENCES

[1]   Srinivasan TM. Genetics, epigenetics, and pregenetics, Int J Yoga. 2011; 4(2): 47–48.
        [http://dx.doi.org/10.4103/0973-6131.85484: 10.4103/0973-6131.85484] [PMID: 22022121]

[2]   EA Mazzio, KF Soliman. Basic concepts of epigenetics: impact of environmental signals on gene expression.Epigenetics. 2012; 7: pp. (2)119-30.
        [http://dx.doi.org/10.4161/epi.7.2.18764] [PMID: 22395460]

[3]   Minocherhomji S, Trygve O.T, Keshav K.S. Mitochondrial regulation of epigenetics and its role in human diseases. Epigenetics 7(4): 326-34.
        [http://dx.doi.org/10.4161/epi.19547]

[4]   Sharma H, Wallace RK. Ayurveda and Epigenetics. Medicine (Baltimore) 2020; 56(12): 687.
        [http://dx.doi.org/10.3390/medicina56120687]

[5]   Sharma S, Kelly TK, Jones PA. Epigenetics in cancer. Carcinogenesis 2010; 31(1): 27-36.
        [http://dx.doi.org/10.1093/carcin/bgp220]

[6]   Sharma H. Ayurveda: Science of life, genetics, and epigenetics, Ayu. 2016; 37(2): 87-91.

[7]   Biémont C. From genotype to phenotype. What do epigenetics and epigenomics tell us? Heredity 2010; 105: 1-3.
[http://dx.doi.org/10.1038/hdy.2010.66]

[8]   Meeran SM, Ahmed A, Tollefsbol TO. Epigenetic targets of bioactive dietary components for cancer prevention and therapy. Clin Epigenetics 2010; 1: 101-16.
[http://dx.doi.org/10.1007/s13148-010-0011-5]

[9]   Rodger EJ, Chatterjee A. The epigenomic basis of common diseases. Clin Epigenetics 2017; 9: 5.
[http://dx.doi.org/10.1186/s13148-017-0313-y]

[10]   Kanherkar RR, Stair SE, Bhatia-Dey N, Mills PJ, Chopra D, Csoka AB. Epigenetic mechanisms of integrative medicine. Evidence-Based Complementary and Alternative Medicine 2017.
[http://dx.doi.org/10.1155/2017/4365429]

CHAPTER 4

The Concept of Prakriti in Perspective of Cancer

Jagruti N. Chaple[1,2,*]

[1] *Department of Kriya Sharir, Mahatma Gandhi Ayurved College, Hospital and Research Centre, Salod (H), Wardha, Maharashtra, India*

[2] *Datta Meghe Institute of Higher Education and Research (DU), Wardha, Maharashtra, India*

Abstract: Currently, there is a lot of talk about cancer (arbuda) at all levels of society. It includes both benign and malignant tumors. Our body is made up of Tridosha, the three fundamental energies or principles that govern our body function on the physical and emotional levels. The three energies are known as Vata, Pitta, and Kapha. Each individual has a different constitution from others. Prakriti is a unique concept of Ayurveda that explains individuality and has a role in maintaining health & prevention, of diseases, and achieving longevity. Each person must know their Prakriti constitution to determine the correct food, exercise, yoga, lifestyle, and environment to remain healthy and achieve longevity. Our Prakriti in Ayurveda roughly resembles DNA or genes in western medicine. Most of the theories offered regarding cancer cause fall into the following categories: embryonic,bio-chemical, infectious agents, and genetic. Ayurveda can play a big role in the last causative factor, genetics. Cancer in each person differs according to the person's exposure to pathogens and Prakriti (genetic constitutions), assessment of Prakriti is very useful in prognosis & therapeutic management of cancer. It is also helpful in prescribing suitable Ahar, Vihar, Yoga & Rasayana therapy.

Keywords: Cancer, Genetic, Prakriti, Tridosha.

INTRODUCTION

Concept of Prakriti: "Prakriti" means "Swabhava," or the nature of the individual. According to Ayurveda, every human being is a separate entity. Prakriti or Bio-typology is an extremely important concept in Ayurveda. Each person is not only different in size and shape, but his physical and psychological character are also different; It is because of predominant panchamahabhuta (five basic elements: Earth, Water, Fire, Air, Space), Dosha (three Bioenergy: Vata, Pitta, Kapha) and Triguna (psychological qualities - Satwa, Rajas, Tamas) at the time of birth which decides their constitution. It is a unique concept of Ayurveda

---

* **Corresponding author Jagruti N. Chaple:** Department of Kriya Sharir Mahatma Gandhi Ayurved College, Hospital and Research Centre, Salod (H), Wardha, Maharashtra, India and Datta Meghe Institute of Higher Education and Research (DU), Wardha, Maharashtra, India; E-mail: chaplejagruti@gmail.com

Vaishali Kuchewar, Gaurav Rajendra Sawarkar, Padam Prasad Simkhada & Mahalaqua Nazli Khatib (Eds.)

that explains individuality and has a role in maintaininghealth, prevention, diagnosis, treatment of diseases, and achieving longevity. Each person must know their constitution to determine the correct food, exercise, yoga, lifestyle, and environment to remain healthy and achieve longevity. We have also explained the way to prevent the disease by selecting proper occupation. Prakriti is formed during the union of sperm and ovum and remains constant for that individual's entire life. It also shows a certain predisposition toward diseases. Hence this concept is also important for physicians.

Prakriti (constitution) assessment is a part of the diagnostic, preventive, and curative methods in the Science of Ayurveda. Ayurveda considers three basic constituents of life classified as three doshas Vata, Pitta, and Kapha. Considering the significant scope of Prakriti, little research has been conducted which highlights the scientific basis of this unique concept of Ayurveda. A few chosen kinds of research are presented here to enlighten the role of the Prakriti concept in modern science. With the help of clinical features of Vata, Pitta and Kapha, we can assess the Prakriti of that person. Hence these seven body types are described on the basis of predominance of doshas present at the time of conception; like the doshaja constitution, the mental constitution is also important. Mental constitution is determined by the relative predominance of Sattva, Raja, and Tama qualities. Sattvic, Rajasik, and Tamasik are the three main constitutions (Table **1**) [1].

ROLE OF PRAKRITI IN THE PATHOGENESIS OF CANCER

A critical review of Samhitas reveal that granthi, arbuda, sarkararbuda, and valmika all indicate different diseases presently known as cancer. Genetics considers DNA as the main constituent of life. Also, the causative factor of the disease in cancer with mutations in DNA. So this creates interest in the search for the application of the philosophy stated by Ayurveda in terms of Modern era of Genetics. Cancer (Arbuda) is muscular swelling that is round, immobile, slightly painful, big, deep-rooted, grows gradually, does not suppurate, and can occur in any part of the body. There are six types of Arbuda described by Acharya Sushruta- 1) Vataja, 2) Pittaj, 3) Kaphaj, 4) Raktaja, 5) Mamsaja, and 6) Medaja. Cancer (Arbuda) forms as a result of the vitiation of Tridosha. Because of changes in dietary habits, lifestyle, pollution, and stress cause vitiation of Doshas and Dhatus. Aggravating factors of Tridosha are –the Vata aggravating factors are excessive intake of Katu, tikta, and kashay Rasas. The Pitta aggravating factors are excessive intake of Amla, Lavan, and Katu Rasas. The Kapha aggravating factors are excessive intake of Madhur, Amla, and Lavan Rasas.

Table 1. Types of Prakriti and appearance.

Kapha Prakriti	Vata Prakriti	Pitta Prakriti

Cancer in each person differs according to the person's exposure to pathogens and person's Prakriti (genetic constitutions), which make each react differently. According to ancient texts, the following are the main factors responsible for the vitiation of Doshas, which may be the causative factor/s in developing a cancer stage.

a. Vata vitiating cause - excessive intake of bitter, pungent, astringent, dry foods and stressful conditions.
b. Vata vitiating causes - excessive intake of sour, salty, fried foods and extreme anger.
c. Kapha vitiating cause- excessive intake of sweet, oily food and sedentary lifestyle.
d. Rakta vitiating causes - excessive intake of acid or alkali-containing foods, fried and roasted foods, alcoholic beverages, extreme anger or severe emotional upset, sunbathing or working under the scorching sun or near the fire and hot conditions, etc. are some other causes
e. Mamsa vitiating causes- excessive use of exudative foods like meat ad some dairy products. Behaviors leading to exudation, like sleeping during the day and overeating, are some of the causes of pathogens invading the fatty tissues.
f. Medo vitiating cause - excessive intake of oily food, sweets, alcohol, and sedentary life.

Other factors causing cancer are cigarette smoking, alcohol, chewing tobacco, and pesticide. The vitiated Dosha vitiates the Mamsa Dhatu at any part of the body, and resulting in metabolic and nutritional derangement. The vitiated Dosha decrease the level of Agni (manifestation of Mandagni), and ultimately Mandagni leads to the formation of Ama. The Agni is present in each cell and is responsible for digestion and metabolic process in the body. The most important active factor in the development of a disease is Ama. Ayurveda does not consider cancer as a separate disease or set of conditions. Instead, Ayurveda states that all diseases are caused due to doshik imbalances and malfunction of Tridosha. Arbuda (Cancer) originates from associations between abnormal bio-factors and weakened body tissues. According to Sushruta Samhita, the Kapha aggravating causative factors such as Guru (Heavy) and Snigdha (Oily) foods, worsen the Kapha and affect the Agni of the body, which result in Mandagni. This leads to improper digestion of food and the formation of Ama, which mix with biological factors and affect the body tissues, changing their qualities. This resulting excessive tissue growth thus forms Cancer (Arbuda).

According to modern medicine, most of the theories have been offered regarding the causes of cancer fall into one of the following categories. 1. Embryonic 2. Bio-chemical 3. Infectious 4. Genetic. Ayurveda can play a big role in genetics. A person's health depends on the 'constitution' with which he is born and how he adapts to his environment. According to Ayurveda, knowledge of the involvement of doshas and dushya is indispensable for prescribing correct therapeutic measures. Epigenetics is the study of how we can change the expression of our genes without altering the sequence of actual DNA or genetic code. Epigenetics is a new field of biology that explores the effects of the environment on cellular behavior. "Environment" includes physical, social, and electromagnetic surroundings, beliefs, perceptions, lifestyles, habits, behaviors, and mental and physical activities. There are two primary and interconnected epigenetic mechanisms - DNA methylation and covalent modification of histone. Many of these processes occur in cancer. Our personality in Ayurveda is similar to our DNA or genes in Western medicine.

Cancer is a genetic disease caused by alterations in the genes and expression of genes. Genetic alterations in most cancers arise in the somatic cells and are transmitted to successive generations of cancer cells but are usually not transferred to the offspring of the patient. However, certain mutations are still an exception for it.If the concept of Panchamahabhoota is applicable, it will differentiate all the particulars present in the cell and change according to the environmental changes as proven. Ayurveda has classified an individual Prakriti on the basis of doshik features which is basic to chose treatment modality in cancer.

SIGNIFICANCE OF PRAKRITI IN VARIOUS CANCER

If Vata constitution person exposed to Vata aggravating factors, it leads to vitiation of Vata causing dushti of Mamsa dhatu, resulted into Arbud.

Similarly, Pitta & Kapha constitution person, if exposed to respective factors may also cause Arbuda manifesting related features. Vitiated Tridosh causes cancer due to dietary changes and lifestyle. Hence, cancer is caused by all three vitiated Dosha, but the more aggravating Dosha is Kapha dosha. Because of excess of Kapha, Cancer (Arbuda) does not suppurate. It is considered as important factor for any growth in the body. Therefore, it is fair to assume that deformed Kapha in the body may be responsible for cancer.

Vata, Pitta & Kapha Prakriti people are more prone to cancer of bone, leukemia or blood cancer & various tumors respectively [2].

Significance of Prakriti assessment:

1. Promotion of health and quality of life and, thereby, longevity.

2. Prevention of disease.

3. Understanding patient needs and risk factors for various chronic conditions.

4. Personalizing health care by monitoring *ahara*, *vihara*, and *aushadhi* individually.

5. Disease management.

6. Reduction in morbidity and mortality.

7. Provision of new approaches for diagnosis and drug development.

8. Reducing the trial and error approach of the health care system.

9. Minimizing adverse drug reactions.

10. Making healthcare affordable for people of various economic strata.

11. To utilize appropriate technologies for developing single and polyherbal products to make them globally acceptable.

PREVENTIVE ASPECTS OF CANCER IN VARIOUS PRAKRITI

The study of Prakriti helps considerably in the treatment of this disease and also:

1. In the patients of cancer, if we assess the Prakriti initially, then the medicines like Shilajit, Amalaki, Haridra as well as Ahara & Vihara can be prescribed which is suitable to particular Prakriti.

2. However, from the point of view of psychology, it is essential to regulate emotional disturbances, particularly Pitta-vitiating ones like anger, anxiety, with the help of some herbs as well as procedures like Shirodhara.

3. Bhallataka (semicarpus Anacardium), Chitraka (Plumbago zeylacica), Aswagandha (Withania somnifera Dunal), and Alarka (Calotropis gigantica) have been reported by many researchers as anti Cancer drugs but these drugs can not be used in every cancer patients. There should be selection of herbs as per the Prakriti of patient i.e. personalize treatment.

4. Therefore Pitta Prakriti cancer patient with the involvement of rakta mamsa dhatu should not prescribed Bhallataka Chitraka. If if necessary, it can be used with low dose using suitable Anupana (vehicle) and Sheetkala (low temperature time in a day).

5. Kapha Prakriti cancer patient with the involvement of medas are better administered with Bhallataka or Chitraka judiciously. Arka (Solanum trilobatum) is considered thridoshahara. As such, it can be administered in all Prakriti without side effects.

6. The same applies to the administration of chemotherapy, radio therapy. As all these are of ushna guna, Pitta Prakriti patient involving pitta sthana like blood, liver, spleen, etc., are to be administered the above therapeutic measures very carefully. The dose and duration of the therapy should to be reduced in the cases of Pitta Prakriti or Pitta predominant disease conditions.

7. Similarly, by prescribing suitable Ahara and Vihara (diet and exercise) and Rasayana drugs, this dreaded disease can be treated and prescribed [3].

Ayurveda is one of the world's oldest health sciences, with core philosophies based on tridosha and Prakriti. These fundamental ideas enable the implementation of methods for not only personalized medicine and treatment but also disease prevention. Various researches are conducted to create scientific evidences for Prakriti (Table **2**).

Table 2. Research studies on prakriti & cancer.

S.N	Title	Authors	Name of Journal
1.	Constitutional study of cancer patients – its Prognostic and therapeutic scope	S.Venkatraghavan, T. P. Sundaresan, V. Rajagopalan & Kanchana Srinivasan	Ancient Science of Life, Vol No. VII No. 2 October 1987, Pages 110 - 115
2	Prakriti and its associations with metabolism, chronic diseases, and genotypes: Possibilities of newborn screening and a lifetime of personalized prevention	Subhodji Dey,Parika Pahava	JAyurveda Integr Med. 2014 Jan-Mar; 5(1): 15–24. doi: 10.4103/0975-9476.128848
3.	Cancer, Inflammation, and Insights from Ayurveda	Venil N. Sumantran, Girish Tillu	Evidence-Based Complementary and Alternative Medicine, vol. 2012, Article ID 306346, 11 pages, 2012. https://doi.org/10.1155/2012/306346
4	Genomic Counterparts to Human Constitution (Prakriti)	Hetal Amin, Rohit Sharma, Mahesh Vyas, Hitesh Vyas	Indian Journal of Ancient Medicine and Yoga Review Article Volume 7 Number 2, April - June 2014
5	Traditional medicine-based therapies for cancer management	Pathirage Kamal Perera	Sys Rev Pharm. 2019;10(1):90-92
6	Prakriti-based medicine: A step towards personalized medicine	Bijoya Chatterjee and Jigisha Pancholi	Ayu. 2011 Apr-Jun; 32(2): 141–146.

CONCLUSION

It is concluded that knowing Prakriti can explain one's ability to fight cancer (Arbuda) because a person who maintains balance in Prakriti is said to have excellent immunity and strength. Disequilibrium in Prakriti greatly increases the threat of Cancer (Arbuda). It is clear from the literary study that Prakriti and Cancer (Arbuda) are closely correlated with each other.

REFERENCES

[1]   Chaple J. Prakriti-important tool for health and disease. J Ind Sys Med 2014; 2(2): 104-06.

[2]   Pooja S, Prasad NB. MB G, Yogesh Kumar P. Correlation of prakriti in prevalence of Cancer (Arbuda). Int J Dev Res 2018; 8(12): 24849-52.

[3]   Venkataraghavan S, Sunderesan TP, Rajagopalan V, Srinivasn K. Constitutional study of cancer patients–its prognostic and therapeutic scope. Anc Sci Life 1987; 7(2): 110.

CHAPTER 5

Screening Tools for Common Cancers

Seema H. Thakare[1,*]

¹ Department of Rognidan and Vikruti Vigyan, Mahatma Gandhi Ayurved College Hospital and Research Centre, Salod (H), Wardha, Maharashtra, India

Abstract: In the present era, because of changing lifestyles and stress, various new diseases are emerging as a major health problem worldwide. Fields like medicine and technology are also getting more advanced, but mortality and morbidity rates are still increasing. In India, after cardiac diseases, cancer is the second leading cause of morbidity and mortality and mainly accounts for 9% of all deaths. Because of a lack of awareness, diagnostic facilities, and screening programs, nearly 75-80% of cancer patients approach hospitals at an advanced stage (stage 3-4). If cancer is detected in the early stage then it is treated easily. Screening is an essential and effective preventive measure in cancer control. The main aim of cancer screening is to detect cancer before the manifestation of symptoms. It is advised for various cancers like breast, cervical, colorectal, prostate, *etc*. Cancer screening is mainly helpful in cancer prevention, early detection, and subsequent treatment. Multiple tools like urine tests, blood tests, medical imaging or DNA tests, *etc*., are mainly used for screening. They help to decrease the total number of people dying of cancer through its early detection and better treatment.

Keywords: Brush biopsy, Colonoscopy, Mammography, Pap smear, Prostate-Specific antigen, Screening tools.

INTRODUCTION

In the present era, there is a huge advancement in the management of cancer, but morbidity and mortality rate is still increasing. As per ICMR's National Cancer Registry Programme, cancer kills more than 1300 Indians daily.

Most cancer patients (75-80%) approach to the hospital in an advanced stage. It might be due to a lack of awareness, lack of diagnostic facilities, and lack of screening programs [1].

---

* **Corresponding author Seema H. Thakare:** Department of Rognidan and Vikruti Vigyan, Mahatma Gandhi Ayurved College Hospital and Research Centre, Salod (H), Wardha, Maharashtra, India; E-mail: seema.thakare@dmimsu.edu.in

Vaishali Kuchewar, Gaurav Rajendra Sawarkar, Padam Prasad Simkhada & Mahalaqua Nazli Khatib (Eds.)

Screening is an essential and effective preventive measure in cancer control. It is one of the components of the national program in India, but still, it has not taken root in most parts of the country [2].

Cancer screening can help to find the disease at the earliest, even before any symptoms start. Cancer may be easy to treat if diagnosed at an early stage.

Up to the 20th century, cancer was diagnosed on the manifestation of its features, and no treatment is effective in such cases [3].

CANCER SCREENING

Cancer screening aims at the early detection of cancer before its manifestation. It is used for various cancers like breast, cervical, colorectal, prostate, *etc.* Urine tests, blood tests, medical imaging or DNA tests, *etc.*, are mainly used for screening.

In the past, cancer screening was usually done for a single organ at a time for high-risk people. Currently, the American cancer society recommends guidelines for population screening. Population screening is recommended for the four most common cancers, *viz.* breast, cervix, colorectal and prostate. It is also known as mass screening or universal screening. It is done without selecting a specific population. While "selective screening" is for high-risk people with a family history of cancer.

However, it is nearly unjustifiable and non-recommended to screen the general population for a maximum of all cancers as no cost-effective intervention is available to detect cancer for a single organ. In contrast, high-risk people can be targeted to increase the prevalence of various single organ cancer types. For example, pancreatic cancer screening can be suggested for those with a strong family history, lung cancer screening may be recommended for those with heavy smoking, and screening for hepatoma is done for people with chronic liver disease. Above mentioned three cancers are the most prevalent and cause maximum deaths in various countries, including the USA. But still, no population-based strategy for screening is used for these cancers [4, 5].

TYPES OF SCREENING TESTS

Each type of cancer has its specific screening test. Following are the screening tests for common types of cancer shown in Table **1**.

Table 1. Screening test for common types of cancer.

S.N	Type of Cancer	Name of Screening Tests
1.	Breast Cancer	1) Breast Self-examination 2) Clinical Breast Examination 3) Mammography 4) Digital Mammography
2.	Cervical Cancer	1) Pap smears 2) Colposcopy 3) Cervicography 4) HPV co-testing
3.	Colorectal Cancer	1) Fecal Occult Blood Testing (FOBT) 2) Stool DNA testing 3) Sigmoidoscopy 4) Colonoscopy 5) Double-Contrast Barium Enema 6) CT Colonography
4.	Prostate Cancer	1) Digital Rectal Examination (DRE) 2) Trans-Rectal Ultrasound (TRUS) 3) Prostate-Specific Antigen (PSA)
5.	Lung Cancer	1) Chest Radiograph 2) Spiral Computed Tomography/Low dose helical (CT or CAT) scan
6.	Oral Cancer	1) Complete Oral Examination 2) Brush Biopsy 3) Toludine blue staining 4) Chemiluminescence 5) Tissue Fluorescence Imaging & Spectroscopy

The detail of the screening is as follows:

Breast Cancer Screening [6, 7]

A) Breast Self-Examination: The patients themselves can perform it. Mainly females of age above 40 years should perform breast self-examination. The patients, while performing breast self-examination, should stand in front of the mirror and perform it. It is the easiest method to identify any breast changes or lumps.

B) Clinical Breast Examination: The method used by the health professional to detect breast lumps or breast changes. Generally, breast examination is used along with mammograms for better diagnosis and results.

C) Mammography: Mammography is the examination of breast tissue with the help of a low dose of x-ray. It is used as a diagnostic as well as a screening tool.

In mammography, the breast tissues were exposed to the radiation in mainly two views, *i.e.* craniocaudal and mediolateral, for a better image of breast tissues.

Mammography should be done every year for women of age 45 to 54 years and every two years for women aged 55 years or more. Mammography has been advanced to digital mode nowadays. Another name for the same is "full-field digital mammography". It is a technique where the solid-state detector is used in place of an x-ray that converts x-ray into electrical signals. It helps patients from being protected from x-ray exposure.

Cervical Cancer Screening [8]

Cervical cancer is the second commonest cancer among the female population in the world. Following various methods are used for cervical cancer screening:

A) Pap Smear Test: It is the mainstay of screening and early detection of cervical cancer. A cervical cell sample is taken with the help of either a wooden or plastic spatula by giving a lithotomy position to the patient. The collected sample is mounted on the glass slide and stained. The cytologist/pathologist then observes the fall under the light microscope for the abnormal cell. The two most common classifications for the Pap smear test results are the Bethesda system and Cervical Intraepithelial Neoplasm (CIN).

B) Colposcopy & Visual Aided Inspection of Cervix: The cervix is visualized with the help of the colposcope or visual aid for detecting any morphological changes in the texture of the cervix. Currently, diluted acetic acid (3%-5%) or Lugol's iodine is applied to the cervix area to detect abnormalities of the cervical part better. The abnormal surface area detected from the caught part of the cervix is then processed for the biopsy.

C) Cervicography: This method was invented in 1981. In this method, 5% diluted acetic acid is applied to the cervix part and pictures are taken with the help of the camera of fixed focal length, and then the expert interprets the photographs.

D) HPV DNA test: The presence of RNA or DNA from carcinogenic Human Papilloma Virus types 16 and 18 in cervical cells is detected by this method. An HPV DNA test is either done by Polymerase chain reaction (PCR) or hybrid capture method (HC).

Colorectal Cancer Screening [9 - 11]

Colorectal cancer (CRC) is one of the most important digestive malignant neoplasms, causing significant mortality and morbidity. Most CRC develops mostly from pre-existing polypoidal growth hence the incidence of CRC can be reduced by endoscopic removal of those polyps.

Following are the screening methods for colorectal cancer:

1) Stool-Based Tests: It is a less invasive and easy method but has to perform repeatedly. If it is positive, the patient is further investigated with the help of a colonoscopy.

A) Fecal Occult Blood Test: It is the preliminary test for suspected colon cancer. In this test, the occult fecal blood is investigated. The origin of blood can not be traced by this method and colonoscopy is required for further diagnosis.

B) Guaiac-based Fecal Occult Test: This test detects hidden, occult blood through the chemical reaction differently than a simple fecal occult blood test. The origin of blood cannot be traced by this method also.

The Stool-based tests should be repeated every three years. If it is found to be positive, the patient is further screened with the help of a colonoscopy.

2. Visual Examination Tests: The colon and rectal structure are visualized, and a biopsy can be performed from the suspected area with this test.

A) Colonoscopy: It is a flexible tube about the width of a half to one centimeter along with a light and small video camera at the end. It is inserted via the anus to the colon. The biopsy from the suspected area or removal of the entire polyp from the colon can be done through colonoscopy. Thus, colonoscopy can be used for screening, diagnosing, treating colonic conditions. For better visualization, the rectum and colon are cleaned with an enema or laxative. The possible complications include a bloated abdomen, low blood pressure, change in the heart rhythm, rupture of the colon or rectum wall, *etc.*

B) CT Colonography: It is also called as Virtual Colonoscopy. Low-dose radiation is used to obtain an internal view of the colon. It is used to screen for polyps or cancers in the large intestine. It is recommended for individuals at increased risk or with a family history of colon cancer. Before colonography, a liquid laxative or enema is given to clear the bowel to visualize the colon properly.

C) Flexible Sigmoidoscopy: Sigmoidoscopy is a thin, flexible tube having light and a very small camera at the end. The preparation of sigmoidoscopy is similar to colonoscopy. It is recommended when a close inspection of the sigmoid colon is required.

Lung Cancer Screening [12]

Lung cancer is very difficult to diagnose at an early stage. For the screening of lung cancer, following tools can be used:

A) Chest Radiograph: Chest radiography was considered an investigating tool used as a screening test for lung carcinoma for many decades because of its wider availability, relatively lower cost and small dose of ionizing radiation. But, chest radiographs failed as the screening tool for lung cancer, mostly detecting lung cancer in advanced stages.

B) Low-dose Helical or Spiral Computed Tomography (CT or CAT) Scan: Low-dose CT was first investigated as a tool for screening lung cancer in Japan then in the USA. It proved a far better tool for screening lung cancer than a chest radiograph and was found to be effective in detecting lung cancer in the initial stages in 84% to 90% of patients. Nowadays, low-dose CT has become widely available for the screening of patients.

Oral Cancer Screening

Oral cancer can be screened through the following methods:

A) Oral Examination: This is the simplest method of screening oral cancer. The dentist or the physician should examine the oral cavity thoroughly for lesions like erythroplakia, leukoplakia, submucosal fibrosis, *etc*.

B) Brush Biopsy: It is also known as the OralCDx brush test. In this test, oral trans-epithelial mucosal sample of cells from the lesion is taken. The non-laceration brush is used for the collection of illustrations and stained with a modified Papanicolaou test. The results are atypical or positive when there is a high suspicion of epithelial dysplasia or carcinoma. When no abnormality is detected, it is labeled as negative.

C) Toluidine Blue Staining: Toluidine blue/Tolonium chloride is a dye used to stain nucleic acids. Hence, it has been widely used for many years as a procedure to identify clinically occult mucosal abnormalities. It is also useful for knowing the extension of cancerous lesions beyond the extent of excision.

D) Chemiluminescence: Clinical examination with chemoluminance has been used to better diagnose the abnormal mucosa in the oral cavity. The patient is asked to rinse the mouth with 1% acetic acid and then wait 1 minute. Then, the patient's oral cavity is examined with the help of chemiluminescent white/blue light. On examination, normal mucosa seems to be blue and abnormal areas show more aceto-white, brighter and distinct margin.

E) Tissue Fluorescence Imaging & Spectroscopy: These are the most recent techniques used to detect oral cancer. Tissue fluorescence imaging and spectroscopy have the advantage of real-time diagnosis and are non-invasive. This technique provides high-resolution images of the oral mucosa's surface and subsurface area to diagnose precancerous and cancerous lesions.

Prostate Cancer Screening [14]

Generally, males above 65 years should be screened for prostate cancer. There is no specific test or tool to screen for prostate cancer. But, the following two tests are widely used to screen for prostate cancer.

A) Digital Rectal Examination (DRE): This is per rectal examination of the prostate gland by the surgeon. A clinically stony hard prostate or the lump in the prostate is considered malignant. But it is not a confirmed tool for screening prostate cancer.

B) Prostate-Specific Antigen (PSA): The blood test called Prostate Specific Antigen (PSA) can be done in suspected cases of prostate cancer. Prostate secretes the Prostate-Specific Antigen (PSA). The normal value of PSA is 0 to 2.5 ng/ml. The level of PSA is increased in prostate cancer. The PSA level may also be grown in various conditions affecting the prostate. So, this test can lack specificity.

CONCLUSION

Modern lifestyles and stress are causing several new ailments worldwide. Due to a lack of awareness, diagnostic facilities, and screening programs, cancer patients arrive at hospitals in severe stages. Early cancer detection simplifies treatment. Screening prevents cancer effectively. Cancer screenings aim to find cancer before it spreads. It is suggested for breast, cervical, colorectal, and prostate cancer. Cancer screening help to prevent, identify and treat the disease in its early stage. Urine, blood, medical imaging, and DNA screenings are prevalent. Early detection and treatment reduce cancer fatalities.

REFERENCES

[1]   Singh M, Prasad CP, Singh TD, Kumar L. Cancer research in India: Challenges & opportunities. Indian J Med Res 2018; 148(4): 362.

[2]   Sahu DP, Subba SH, Giri PP. Cancer awareness and attitude towards cancer screening in India: A narrative review. J Family Med Prim Care 2020; 9(5): 2214.

[3]   Wardle J, Robb K, Vernon S, Waller J. Screening for prevention and early cancer diagnosis. Am Psychol 2015; 70(2): 119.

[4]   Ahlquist DA. Universal cancer screening: revolutionary, rational, and realizable. NPJ Precis Oncol 2018; 2(1): 1-5.

[5]   Wilson JM, Jungner G. Principles and practice of screening for disease. World Health Organization 1968.

[6]   Elmore JG, Armstrong K, Lehman CD, Fletcher SW. Screening for breast cancer. JAMA 2005; 293(10): 1245-56.

[7]   Smith RA, Saslow D, Sawyer KA, *et al.* American Cancer Society guidelines for breast cancer screening: update 2003. CA Cancer J Clin 2003; 53(3): 141-69.

[8]   Misiri H. Cervical cancer screening methods. Research 2014.

[9]   Available from: https://www.cancer.org/cancer/colon-rectal-cancer/detection-diagnosis-staging.html

[10]   Walsh JM, Terdiman JP. Colorectal cancer screening: scientific review. JAMA 2003; 289(10): 1288-96.

[11]   Triantafillidis JK, Vagianos C, Gikas A, Korontzi M, Papalois A. Screening for colorectal cancer: the role of the primary care physician. Eur J Gastroenterol Hepatol 2017; 29(1): e1-7.

[12]   Kanne JP. Screening for lung cancer: what have we learned? AJR Am J Roentgenol 2014; 202(3): 530-5.

[13]   Fedele S. Diagnostic aids in the screening of oral cancer. Head Neck Oncol 2009; 1(1): 1-6.

[14]   Descotes JL. Diagnosis of prostate cancer. Asian J Urol 2019; 6(2): 129-36.

CHAPTER 6

Herbs for Cancer

Akshay Sudhir Pargaonkar[1,*], Bharat Rathi[2] and Bhagyashree R. Jibkate[2]

[1] *Department of Dravyaguna Vigyan, Mahatma Gandhi Ayurved, College Hospital & Research Centre, Salod (H), Wardha, Maharashtra, 442001, India*

[2] *Department of Rasashastra & Bhaishajya Kalpana, Mahatma Gandhi Ayurved College Hospital & Research Centre, Salod (H), Wardha, Maharashtra, 442001, India*

Abstract: In the present era of modernization, the new generation differs from the lifestyle maintained in the ancient period. A few decades ago, it was a regular practice of major community, *i.e.*, Early to bed and early to rise, where the body's clock and nature's clock were more or less similar. During this period of modernization, there was a tremendous change in lifestyle, including daily activities. This results in an early facing of severe problems. Modern medicines very well deal with such issues, but long-term regular use of such medication can affect vital organs in the future. Medicinal herbs have been used worldwide as supportive treatment to minimize the toxic effects of chemotherapy and radiotherapy. Many clinical studies have reported the beneficial results of herbs in combination with conventional therapeutics on the patients' survival, immune modulation, and quality of life. One such disease is cancer, wherein medicines have various side effects and immunity suppression effects. The present chapter deals with different herbs, their role in cancer treatment, and the side effects of their treatment. Here in this chapter, herbs are briefly reviewed that are used for treating various cancers. Different research work and clinical studies are mentioned here that showed the anticancer activities and their effect on various biological pathways. The use of a dietary regime along with medicinal herbs for better results is also a part of Ayurveda to be followed. The state of balance between doshas and dhatus is essential while using herbs in all aspects. This review may help to provide the utility of various herbs in various aspects of cancer and its treatment.

Keywords: Ayurveda herbs, Cancer, Chemotherapy, Radiotherapy.

INTRODUCTION

This chapter is devoted to the herbs which can be used to prevent cancer as a support in the treatment and to minimize the side effects of chemotherapy and radiotherapy.

---

[*] **Corresponding author Akshay Sudhir Pargaonkar:** Department of Dravyaguna Vigyan, Mahatma Gandhi Ayurved College Hospital & Research Centre, Salod (H), Wardha, Maharashtra, 442001, India; Email: akshay.pargaonkar@dmimsu.edu.in

Vaishali Kuchewar, Gaurav Rajendra Sawarkar, Padam Prasad Simkhada & Mahalaqua Nazli Khatib (Eds.)

Following medicines have the potential against cancer.

Ashwagandha (*Withania somnifera* (Linn.) Dunal)

It is a flowering plant of the Solanaceae family. *It* is *Katu, Tikta Kashaya rasatmak, Katuvipak*, and *Ushnaveeryatmak*. There are 23 varieties of Withania in which only *W. somnifera* and *W. coagulance* are medicinally important. The root of *W. somnifera* is used for medicinal purposes. *W. somnifera* has 12 alkaloids, 35 withanolides, and several other sitoindosides. These compounds proved to act in apoptosis, angiogenesis, anti-inflammatory, immune response, stress response, and effectiveness against cancer [1]. Some studies showed that *W. somnifera* might reduce the growth of the tumor without damaging the normal cell. It has sedative effects and interferes with certain chemotherapy drugs [2]. It should be used cautiously in breast and prostate cancer as it can elevate DHEA and increase testosterone. Some researchers also show interference in the immunoassay of serum digoxin level measurement [3].

Guduchi (*Tinospora cordifolia* (Wild) Miers)

It is a deciduous, large climbing shrub of the Menispermaceae family and is distributed in tropical regions of India. Leaves are simple, alternate, and heart-shaped with long petioles. The most common part used for medicinal purposes is the stem and leaves. Still, its roots also contain many important and useful alkaloids. *T. cordifilia* helps to alleviate *Vata* and *Kapha* dosha and is also very beneficial in *raktaj vyadhi*. In *Ayurveda*, it is called *Amruta* for its capability to enhance vitality and longevity. *T. cordifolia* normalizes biological processes like proliferation, apoptosis, lipid metabolism, *etc.* by activating the human lymphocyte with the synthesis of Pro-inflammatory cytokines like TNF- α, interleukin beta (IL-1b), interleukin (IL-6,) IL-18, interferon's (IFN-c) [4]. T. cordifolia also reduces oxidative stress by increasing the tissue glycoprotein [5]. Glucosides, Glycoside, and alkaloids of *T. cordifilia* inhibits NF-KB and acts as a nitric oxide scavenger, proving its action against cancer. It also shows a chemo-radio protective role by improving patients' body weight, tissue weight, and tubular diameter. This herb's antioxidant and immunomodulatory properties also help protect during chemo or radiation therapy.

Kalmegh (Andrographis paniculata (Burm. F.) Nees)

Andrographis paniculata is a small annual herb belonging to the Acanthaceae family. Stem weak, and flowers are small, white, or purple colored. Fruits are small and round and contain pale brown seeds. Flowering and fruiting are seen from the spring season to the summer season. Plant extract shows anti-inflammatory, analgesic, immune enhancer, hepatoprotective, and anticancer activities. Phytochemical compounds like Andrographolide and Neoandro-grapholide inhibit LPS and PGE2 synthesis and have potential cell differentiation-inducing activity on leukemia cells [6]. Flavonoids, quercetin, genistein, and baicalein derived from plant extracts show anti-tumor effects. The study shows increased proliferation of lymphocytes and production of IL-2 by the action of immunostimulatory activity of andrographolide. It also improved the factor of tumor necrosis α production and CD markers, increasing the cytotoxic activity against cancer cells [7].

Haridra (*Curcuma longa* Linn.)

Curcuma longa is a well-known herb widely used in *Ayurveda*. It is a perennial herbaceous plant having smooth, alternate, green, and tapering. The rhizomes of this plant are used for medicinal purposes, are cylindrical, and have a strong aroma. In practice, *C. longa* has received considerable attention for its antiseptic, analgesic, antioxidant, anti-inflammatory, and anticancer activities. This drug acts as an anticancer drug by causing mutagenesis, cell cycle regulation, apoptosis, and oncogene expression. *C. longa* acts on various biological pathways. The study shows the action of anticancer activities *via* its effect on various biological pathways responsible for apoptosis, cell cycle regulation, mutagenesis, tumorigenesis, oncogene expression, and metastasis. Curcumin inhibits NF-kB, and downstream gene products (including c-myc, Bcl-2, COX-2, NOS, Cyclin D1, TNF-α, interleukins, and MMP-9) also act as an antiproliferative in multiple malignancies. Curcumin is the main compound of *C. longa,* the principal curcuminoid. Neutralizing lipid radicals has resulted from the chain-breaking antioxidant action of curcumin. In the initial stage of carcinoma, free radicles and antioxidant properties of *C. longa* plays a major role. The study shows the UV irradiation suppression activity, regulation of pro-angiogenic growth factor, bFGF, VEGF, angiopoietin 1, 2 COX -2, matrix metalloproteinase-9(MMP-9), AP-1, and NF-κB responsible for carcinogenic effects. Curcumin stimulates DDR (DNA damage response) as a chemopreventive agent. By reversing the bile acid suppression of gene expression SOD-1, the herb shows chemoprotective effects in an effective esophageal cell exposed to bile acid [8 - 10].

Neem (Azadirachta indica Linn.)

Azadirachta indica is an evergreen tree that belongs to the Meliaceae family. The tree has simple opposite leaves short – straight trunk with white fragment flowers found in tropical and subtropical regions of India. This herb contains various compounds like Nimbin, nimbinine, azadiractole, azadirachtin, nimbadinol, β-sitosterol, *etc.* bioactive components of *A. indica,* such as azadirachtin, nimbolid, *etc.*, which show chemopreventive and anti-tumor effects. *A. indica* shows inhibition of cell proliferation through the disruption of cell cycle progression, suppression of angiogenesis, cellular reduction restoration and enhancement of immune response against carcinogens. Extracting *A. indica* reduces the DNA mutation and improves genome stability; it increases O6-methylguanine-DNA methyltransferase on a cellular level with demethylation activity in peripheral blood lymphocytes and cancer cells. Reduction of excessive proliferation, restoration of cellular redox balance, inhibition of angiogenesis, stimulation of cell death, and enhancement of immune response are the main actions for which *A. indica* is used as an anticancer drug [11, 12].

Sadabahar/Sadapushpa (Vinca rosea Linn.)

Vinca rosea is a species of flowering plant of the Apocynaceae family. It is an evergreen sub-shrub having oval, broad, glossy green leaves with a pale midrib and short petiole. Flowers are white to dark pink colored with five petals. Certain chemical components like vinblastine, vincristine catharanthine, vindoline, vinorelbine, vinculin, Rosinidin, and Lochnericine are found in *V. rosea*. Alkaloids from *V. rosea* are important as they produce anticancer effects [13]. Vinblastine slows down angiogenesis or the formation of new vessels in malignancy. Sometimes it may cause angina or secretion of antidiuretic hormone. Vinorelbine performs the same action as vinblastine. It slows down the growth of breast cancer tumors and shows anti-proliferation action on osteosarcoma. It decreases the stability of the lipid bilayer membrane. Vinorelbine may cause constipation, nausea, bleeding, numbness, or tingling. Vincristine has a powerful inhibition action against microtubule formation. Vindesine has the same effect as vinblastine. But it may cause toxicity of blood cells, malaise, tingling, and anemia in some cases. The route of administration for all four alkaloids is intravenous. These alkaloids are used with a combination of chemotherapy regimens for medicinal therapy. These alkaloids arrest cell division and cause cell death through their cytotoxic effects [14].

Adrak/Shunthi (Zingiber officinale)

Zinziber officinale is a perennial herb found widely in tropical Asia. The leaves of this plant are pointed and lanceolate. The stem is leafy and thick. Its rhizome is used for medicinal purposes: tuberous, fleshy, and aromatic. This plant contains a-curumene, B-D-curumene, B- bourbornene, d- Borneal, D- camphene, Geraniol, Gingerol, a & b – zingiberenes, Zingiberol, Zingiberon, Gingerone A, Gingerdiol, Gingerone B & C. These compounds block the elevated NFκB, TNF-α, pro-inflammatory cytokine, *etc.*, and prove effective in cancer. Activated TNF α genes release pro-inflammatory cytokines, which cause activation of NFκB; it results in the activation of other inflammatory cytokines such as COX-2, LOX-2, chemokines, and iNOS, which initiates carcinogenesis. The study showed effective results of *Z. officinale* against gastric cancer, pancreatic, liver, colorectal, and cholangiocarcinoma [15].

Tulsi (Ocimum sanctum)

O. sanctum is one of the important sources of medicine or drug. This plant belongs to the Lamiaceae family and grows in tropical and warm areas. Leaves are aromatic. Flowers are small, purple-colored, with small fruits having reddish-yellow seeds. Two varieties of *O. sanctum* are used for medicinal purposes Krushna tulsi and Rama tulsi. *O. sanctum* contains active components like eugenol, rosmarinic, apigenin, luteolin, myretenal, carnosic, and β systesterol. These compounds block the action of COX 2 and prevent inflammation and pain. A compound like eugenol reduces the division and migration of malignant cells and induces apoptosis by preventing the attack of cancer cell on the surrounding structure. Compounds such as eugenol, rosmarinic, apigenin, luteolin, myretenal, carnosic, and β systesterol destroy the malignant cells by their antioxidant activity. These compounds block the proliferation and prevent angiogenesis. Many studies showed its efficacy in skin, lung, breasts, prostate, liver, stomach, and oral cancer [16 - 19].

Amalaki (*Emblica officinalis* Gaertn)

It is a medium-sized tree that belongs to the Euphorbiaceae family. Leaves are simple, pinnate, tiny, and closely set along the branchlets. Flowers are yellow, fruits are smooth cylindrical and have six vertical stripes. *E. officinalis* possess phytochemicals like pyrogallol, gallic acid, ellagic acid phytochemicals, norsesquiterpenoids, corilagin, elaeocarpusin, geraniin, prodelphinidins B1 and B2. *E. officinalis* has chemopreventive, antioxidant, free radical screening, anti-inflammatory, antimutagenic, and immunomodulatory properties useful in managing cancer. Some prophylaxis studies showed that the genotoxic effects of heavy metals and carcinogen benzopyrene are reduced after the consumption of *E. officinalis*. Some reflections on skin carcinogenesis showed that the continuous administration of *E. officinalis* reduced the incidence of the tumor by 60% ellagic acid, gallic acid, chebulagic acid, and some other tannins, preventing lipid peroxidation and mutagenesis in response to carcinogens [20 - 22].

Inhibition of NF- kappa B results in persistent apoptosis and is also an important factor for survival in cancer cell. This tennis, including ellagic acid, gallic acid, chebulagic acid, *etc.*, restricts the inhibition of NF-kappaB and acts as an antiproliferative and proapoptotic. Various studies showed that the phytoconstituents of *E. officinalis* are effective in cancers of the colon, prostate, and breast [23 - 25].

Bhumyamalaki (Phyllanthus amarus Schum & Thonn)

It is a tropical weed that grows in moist sunny places and belongs to the phyllanthaceae family. It has small tiny capsule fruits and pale green flowers. *P. amarus* contain various phytoconstituents like steroidal hormone, flavonoids, triterpenes, *etc.* Various studies showed its potent anti-carcinogenic activities in various models. Potent antiproliferative activities are seen in the methanolic extract of *P. amarus*. *It* showed antimetastatic action by inducing apoptosis. Polyphenol compounds of *P. amarus* extract also prove its antimetastatic activities and inhibition of cell cycle regulators and DNA repair [26 - 28].

HERBS TO NEUTRALIZE THE TOXICITY OF CHEMOTHERAPY & RADIOTHERAPY

Chemotherapy and radiotherapy are the mainstay of treatment to kill malignant cells or reduce their size and stop them from spreading. It affects normal cells in the body, like skin, bone marrow, mucosa, hairs, nails, blood cells, *etc.*

According to *Ayurveda*, cell division or cell proliferation is caused by the aggravation of *Vata dosha* and the inhibition of *Kapha dosha*. Most of the side effects of chemo-radiotherapy can be correlated with the symptoms of aggravated Pitta dosha like *asyavipaka* (stomatitis), *raktapitta* (hemorrhage), *sheetapitta* (urticaria), *Daha* (burning sensation in body), *ushmadhikya* (increase in body temperature), *khalitya* (alopecia), *chardi* (vomiting), *etc.* and features of vitiation of *Vata* and *kaphashwetavabhasta* (pallor), *udardashool* (abdominal pain), *path* (tremors), *padasuptata* (numbness of foot), *ucchashruti* (hearing loss), *nakhabheda* (cracking nails), *etc.* (Tables **1** and **2**).

Following herbs are studied for their efficacy in reducing the adverse effect of cancer treatment.

Zingiber officinale

Various studies show tissue-protective, radioprotective, antioxidant, and immunostimulant activities of extracts of *Z. officinale*. A study shows a reduction effect of hydrochloric extract of *Z. officinale* in the severity of radiation sickness and mortality [8]. Because of its antioxidant, neuromodulatory, and radioprotective mechanism, *Z. officinale* acts as a gastroprotective agent in radiation.

Allium Satiivum Linn

Immuno modulatory and antioxidant mechanism shows their anticancer and chemoprotective activities. Protein lactins or ASA I and II of *A. sattivum* have immunomodulatory effects and mitogenetic action towards murine splenocytes, thymocytes, human peripheral blood lymphocytes, *etc.* Organosulfur compounds like diallyl sulfide (DAS), diallyl disulfide (DADS), s-ethyl cysteine (SEC), and n-ethyl cysteine from *A. sattivum* show antioxidant effects and protect against lipid oxidations [29].

Semicarpus Anacardium Linn.f.

K-40 compound of *S. anacardium* shows effective radioprotective activity [29]. This potentiates the efficiency of anticancer drugs like mitomycin-c, 5- flurouracil and methotrexate. This herb also detoxifies hepatocarcinogenesis and aflatoxin B1 [30].

Phyllanthus Amarus Schum & Thonn

Reduction in myelosuppression and increase in WBC, cellularity of bone marrow, and maturation of monocytes report its chemoprotective activity. *P. amarus* showed good anticancer and hepatoprotective activity against 20 MC and aflatoxin B (1) [28].

Punica Granatum Linn

Many studies on *P.granatum showed its activity of c*ell cycle disruption, apoptosis, anti-proliferation, and inhibition of tumor growth. Similarly, antioxidants and flavonoids present in *P. granatum* showed their radioprotective action [29].

Ocimum Sanctum Linn

O. sanctum proved to be anti-angiogenic, antiproliferative, and pro-apoptosis in prostate cancer and also shows radioprotective and chemoprotective effects [30].

Boerrhavia Diffusa Linn

This antioxidant and immunomodulatory drug shows anti-proliferation and apoptosis activities against cervical cancer. This herb normalizes cytokine production and triggers the cell immune system [31].

Table 1. List of some herbs to eliminate adverse effects during or after chemo/radiotherapy.

Herb	Uses	Useful Part
Bilva	Promotes normal digestive health and is effective in diarrhea.	Leaves, Fruits
Amalaki	Promotes normal digestive health and effective in diarrhea.	Raw & dried fruits

(Table 1) cont.....

Herb	Uses	Useful Part
Haritaki	Constipation	Fruits
Jatamansi	Sleeplessness	Roots
Bala	Fatigue, weakness	Root, Bark, Leaves, Flowers, Seeds.
Brahmi, Haritaki, Vacha	Useful in memory decline.	*Brahmi* – whole plant *Haritaki* – Fruits *Vacha* - Rhizome
Bhringaraj, Brahmi	Useful in hair loss.	Roots, Whole plant
Shatavari	Supports and normalizes digestion, helpful in stomach ulcer, inflammatory, and menopausal conditions. Promotes rejuvenation of tissues.	Roots
Guduchi	Balances tridosha, protects WBC, improves and builds up the body's defense mechanism, and prevents infection.	Leaves, Bark, Stem.
Triphala	Increases RBCs, balances tridosha, promotes normal appetite, nourishes, and rejuvenates tissue.	Fruits

Table 2. List of herbs used for their anticancer and chemoprotective activities.

Sr. No.	Drug	Botanical Name	Useful Part	*Rasa Panchak*
1.	*Adraka*	*Zingiber officinale*	Rhizome	*Rasa-Katu Guna-Tikshna, Guru, Ruksha Virya-Ushna Vipaka-Madhur* Action on dosha– Balances *Kapha dosha.*
Research work done				

Research work done

1.Habib SH, Makpol S, Hamid NA, Das S, Ngah WZ, Yusof YA. Ginger extract (*Zingiber officinale*) has anticancer and anti-inflammatory effects on ethionine-induced hepatoma rats. Clinics. 2008;63(6):807-13.

2. Sang S, Hong J, Wu H, Liu J, Yang CS, Pan MH, Badmaev V, Ho CT. Increased growth inhibitory effects on human cancer cells and anti-inflammatory potency of shogaols from *Zingiber officinale* relative to gingerols. Journal of agricultural and food chemistry. 2009 Nov 25;57(22):10645-50.

3. Liu Y, Whelan RJ, Pattnaik BR, Ludwig K, Subudhi E, Rowland H, Claussen N, Zucker N, Uppal S, Kushner DM, Felder M. Terpenoids from *Zingiber officinale* (Ginger) induce apoptosis in endometrial cancer cells through the activation of p53. PloS one. 2012 Dec 31;7(12):e53178.

Hickok JT, Roscoe JA, Morrow GR, Ryan JL. A phase II/III randomized, placebo-controlled, double-blind clinical trial of ginger (Zingiber officinale) for nausea caused by chemotherapy for cancer: a currently accruing URCC CCOP Cancer Control Study. Supportive cancer therapy. 2007 Sep 1;4(4):247-50.

5. Abdullah S, Abidin SA, Murad NA, Makpol S, Ngah WZ, Yusof YA. Ginger extract (Zingiber officinale) triggers apoptosis and G0/G1 cell arrest in HCT 116 and HT 29 colon cancer cell lines. African Journal of Biochemistry Research. 2010 May 31;4(5):134-42.

(Table 2) cont.....

Sr. No.	Drug	Botanical Name	Useful Part	Rasa Panchak
2.	*Amalaki*	*Emblica officinalis* Gaerth.	Raw & dried fruits	*Rasa- Pancha rasatmak* *Guna-Guru, Sheeta* *Virya-Sheeta* *Vipaka-Madhur* Action on dosha – Balances all three *doshas*
Research work done	1. Baliga MS, Dsouza JJ. Amla (*Emblica officinalis* Gaertn) is a wonder berry in cancer treatment and prevention. European Journal of Cancer Prevention. 2011 May 1;20(3):225-39. 2. Vadde R, Radhakrishnan S, Kurundu HE, Reddivari L, Vanamala JK. Indian gooseberry (*Emblica officinalis* Gaertn.) suppresses cell proliferation and induces apoptosis in human colon cancer stem cells independent of p53 status *via* suppression of c-Myc and cyclin D1. Journal of Functional Foods. 2016 Aug 1;25:267-78. 3. Haque R, Bin-Hafeez B, Ahmad I, Parvez S, Pandey S, Raisuddin S. Protective effects of *Emblica officinalis* Gaertn. in cyclophosphamide-treated mice. Human & experimental toxicology. 2001 Dec;20(12):643-50. 4. JOSE JK, KUTTAN G, GEORGE J, KUTTAN R. Antimutagenic and anti-carcinogenic activity of *Emblica officinalis* Gaertn. Journal of clinical biochemistry and nutrition. 1997;22(3):171-6. 5. Nandi P, Talukder G, Sharma A. Dietary chemoprevention of clastogenic effects of 3, 4-benzo (a) pyrene by *Emblica officinalis* Gaertn. Fruit extract. British journal of cancer. 1997 Nov;76(10):1279-83.			
3.	*Arka*	*Calotropis procera*	Leaves, Latex, Flowers, Root	*Rasa-K-T* *Guna-Laghu, Ruksha* *Virya -Ushna* *Vipaka -Katu* Action on dosha - Balances *Vata* and *Kapha*
Research work done	1. de Oliveira JS, Bezerra DP, de Freitas CD, Marinho Filho JD, de Moraes MO, Pessoa C, Costa-Lotufo LV, Ramos MV. *In vitro* cytotoxicity against different human cancer cell lines of laticifer proteins of *Calotropis Procera* (Ait.) R. Br. Toxicology *in vitro*. 2007 Dec 1;21(8):1563-73. 2. Samy RP, Rajendran P, Li F, Anandi NM, Stiles BG, Ignacimuthu S, Sethi G, Chow VT. Identify a novel *Calotropis procera* protein that can suppress tumor growth in breast cancer by suppressing the NF-κB pathway. PloS one. 2012 Dec 20;7(12):e48514. 3. Verma SK, Singh SK, Mathur A. *In vitro* cytotoxicity of *Calotropis Procera* and Trigonella foenum-graecum against human cancer cell lines. J Chem Pharm Res. 2010;2(2):861-165. 4. Mathur R, Gupta SK, Mathur SR, Velpandian T. Anti-tumor studies with extracts of *Calotropis Procera* (Ait.) R. Br. root employing Hep2 cells and their possible mechanism of action. 5. Choedon T, Mathan G, Arya S, Kumar VL, Kumar V. Anticancer and cytotoxic properties of the latex of *Calotropis Procera* in a transgenic mouse model of hepatocellular carcinoma. World Journal of Gastroenterology: WJG. 2006 Apr 28;12(16):2517.			

(Table 2) cont.....

Sr. No.	Drug	Botanical Name	Useful Part	*Rasa Panchak*
4.	*Ashoka*	*Saraca asoka* Roxb DC	Bark, Flowers, Seeds.	*Rasa-Kashay, Tikta* *Guna -Laghu, Ruksha* *Virya -Sheeta* *Vipaka -Katu* Action on dosha - Balance *Kapha* and *Pitta dosha.*
Research work done	1. Cibin TR, Devi DG, Abraham A. Chemoprevention of skin cancer by the flavonoid fraction of Saraca asoka. Phytotherapy Research: An International Journal Devoted to Pharmacological and Toxicological Evaluation of Natural Product Derivatives. 2010 May;24(5):666-72. 2. Cibin TR, Devi DG, Abraham A. Chemoprevention of two-stage skin cancer *in vivo* by Saraca asoca. Integrative Cancer Therapies. 2012 Sep;11(3):279-86. 3. Yadav NK, Saini KS, Hossain Z, Omer A, Sharma C, Gayen JR, Singh P, Arya KR, Singh RK. *Saraca indica* bark extract shows *in vitro* antioxidant and anti-breast cancer activity and does not exhibit toxicological effects. Oxidative medicine and cellular longevity. 2015 Jan 1;2015. 4. Lin JK, Tsai SH. Chemoprevention of cancer and cardiovascular disease by resveratrol. Proceedings of the National Science Council, Republic of China. Part B, Life sciences. 1999 Jul 1;23(3):99-106.			
5.	*Ashwagandha*	*Withania somnifera* Dunal.	Leaves, Root	*Rasa- K-T- Kaashay* *Guna- Snigdha, Laghu,* *Virya- Ushna* *Vipaka- Katu* Action on dosha- Balances tridosha especial *Kapha* and *vata*
Research Work done	1. Biswal BM, Sulaiman SA, Ismail HC, Zakaria H, Musa KI. Effect of *Withania somnifera* (*Ashwagandha*) on developing chemotherapy-induced fatigue and quality of life in breast cancer patients. Integrative cancer therapies. 2013 Jul;12(4):312-22. 2. Achar GP, Prabhakar BT, Rao S, George T, Abraham S, Sequeira N, Baliga MS. Scientific Validation of the Usefulness of *Withania somnifera* Dunal in the Prevention and Treatment of Cancer. InAnticancer Plants: Properties and Application 2018 (pp. 285-301). Springer, Singapore. 3. Kaur K, Widodo N, Nagpal A, Kaul SC, Wadhwa R. Sensitization of human cancer cells to anticancer drugs by leaf extract of *Ashwagandha* (Lash). Tissue Culture Research Communications. 2007;26(4):193-9. 4. Madhuri S, Govind P. Anticancer activity of *Withania somnifera* Dunal (*Ashwagandha*). Indian Drugs. 2009;46(8):603-9. 5. Mehta V, Chander H, Munshi A. Mechanisms of Anti-Tumor Activity of *Withania somnifera* (*Ashwagandha*). Nutrition and Cancer. 2020 Jun 13:1-3.			
6.	*Bhallataka*	*Semecarpus anacardium* Linn.	Seeds, Fruits	*Rasa-K-T-Kashay* *Guna Laghu,Teekshna,Snigdha* *Virya -Ushna* *Vipaka -Madhur* Action on dosha -Balances *Kapha dosha*

Sr. No.	Drug	Botanical Name	Useful Part	*Rasa Panchak*
Research work done	1. Mathivadhani P, Shanthi P, Sachdanandam P. Apoptotic effect of *Semecarpus anacardium* nut extract on T47D breast cancer cell line. Cell biology international. 2007 Oct;31(10):1198-206. 2. Veena K, Shanthi P, Sachdanandam P. The biochemical alterations following administration of Kalpaamruthaa and *Semecarpus anacardium* in mammary carcinoma. Chemical-biological interactions. 2006 May 15;161(1):69-78. 3. Patel SR, Suthar AP, Patel RM. *In vitro* cytotoxicity activity of *Semecarpus anacardium* extract against Hep 2 and Vero cell lines. Int J PharmTech Res. 2009 Oct;1:1429-33. 4. Premalatha B, Sachdanandam P. Potency of *Semecarpus Anacardium* Linn. nut milk extracts against aflatoxin B1-induced hepatocarcinogenesis: reflection on microsomal biotransformation enzymes. Pharmacological Research. 2000 Aug 1;42(2):161-6.			
7.	*Bhumyamalaki*	*Phyllanthus niruri* sensu. Hook F	Whole plant	Rasa-T-Kashay-Madhur Guna-Lagu, Ruksha Virya-Sheeta *Vipaka-Madhur* Action on dosha - *Kapha pitta shamak*
Research work done	1. Sharma P, Parmar J, Verma P, Sharma P, Goyal PK. Anti-tumor activity of *Phyllanthus niruri* (a medicinal plant) on chemical-induced skin carcinogenesis in mice. Asian Pac J Cancer Prev. 2009 Jan 1;10(6):1089-94. 2. Unni RT, Shah GA, Snima KS, Kamath CR, Nair SV, Lakshmanan VK. Enhanced delivery of *Phyllanthus niruri* nanoparticles for prostate cancer therapy. Journal of Bionanoscience. 2014 Apr 1;8(2):101-7. 3. Júnior RF, Soares LA, da Costa Porto CR, de Aquino RG, Guedes HG, Petrovick PR, de Souza TP, Araújo AA, Guerra GC. Growth inhibitory effects of *Phyllanthus niruri* extracts in combination with cisplatin on cancer cell lines. World Journal of Gastroenterology: WJG. 2012 Aug 21;18(31):4162. 4. Lee SH, Jaganath IB, Wang SM, Sekaran SD. Antimetastatic effects of Phyllanthus on human lung (A549) and breast (MCF-7) cancer cell lines. PloS one. 2011 Jun 16;6(6):e20994.			
8.	*Bilva*	*Aegle marmelos* Linn Conr.	Fruits Ripen fruit Unripe fruit	*Rasa-K-T-Kashay Guna-Grahi,Snigdha, Tikta Virya-Ushna Vipaka-Katu* Action on dosha - Balances *Tridosha*

(Table 2) cont.....

Sr. No.	Drug	Botanical Name	Useful Part	*Rasa Panchak*
Research work done	1. Baliga MS, Thilakchand KR, Rai MP, Rao S, Venkatesh P. *Aegle marmelos* (L.) Correa (Bael) and its phytochemicals in the treatment and prevention of cancer. Integrative cancer therapies. 2013 May;12(3):187-96. 2. Arora D, Sharma N, Singamaneni V, Sharma V, Kushwaha M, Abrol V, Guru S, Sharma S, Gupta AP, Bhushan S, Jaglan S. Isolation and characterization of bioactive metabolites from Xylaria psidii, an endophytic fungus of the medicinal plant *Aegle marmelos* and their role in mitochondrial-dependent apoptosis against pancreatic cancer cells. Phytomedicine. 2016 Nov 15;23(12):1312-20. 3. Bhatti R, Singh J, Saxena AK, Suri N, Ishar MP. Pharmacognostic standardization and antiproliferative activity of *Aegle marmelos* (L.) Correa is leaves in various human cancer cell lines. Indian journal of pharmaceutical sciences. 2013 Nov;75(6):628. 4. Subramaniam D, Giridharan P, Murmu N, Shankaranarayanan NP, May R, Houchen CW, Ramanujam RP, Balakrishnan A, Vishwakarma RA, Anant S. Activation of apoptosis by 1-hydroxy-5, 7-dimethoxy-2-naphthalene-carboxaldehyde, a novel compound from Aegle marmelos. Cancer Research. 2008 Oct 15;68(20):8573-81. 5. Seemaisamy R, Faruck LH, Gattu S, Neelamegam R, Bakshi HA, Rashan L, Al-Buloshi M, Hasson SS, Nagarajan K. Anti-microbial and anti-cancer activity of *Aegle Marmelos* And gas chromatography coupled spectrometry analysis of their chemical constituents. International Journal of Pharmaceutical Sciences and Research. 2019 Jan 1;10(1):373-80.			
9.	*Chandan*	*Santalum album* Linn.	Wood, oil	*Rasa -T-M* *Guna -Laghu,Ruksha* *Virya -Sheeta* *Vipaka -Katu* Action on dosha - Balances *Kapha Pitta dosha*
Research work done	1. Kim TH, Ito H, Hatano T, Takayasu J, Tokuda H, Nishino H, Machiguchi T, Yoshida T. New anti-tumor sesquiterpenoids from *Santalum album* of Indian origin. Tetrahedron. 2006 Jul 17;62(29):6981-9. 2. Santha S, Dwivedi C. Anticancer effects of sandalwood (*Santalum album*). Anticancer Research. 2015 Jun 1;35(6):3137-45. 3. Kavithaa K, Paulpandi M, Ponraj T, Murugan K, Sumathi S. Induction of intrinsic apoptotic pathway in human breast cancer (MCF-7) cells through facile biosynthesized zinc oxide nanorods. Karbala International Journal of Modern Science. 2016 Mar 1;2(1):46-55.			
10.	*Chirayata*	*Smertia chirata* Buch Ham	Whole plant	*Rasa -Tikta* *Guna -Laghu, Ruksha* *Virya -Sheeta* *Vipaka -Katu* Action on dosha - Balances *Kapha and Pitta*

(Table 2) cont.....

Sr. No.	Drug	Botanical Name	Useful Part	*Rasa Panchak*
Research work done	\multicolumn{4}{l}{}

Sr. No.	Drug	Botanical Name	Useful Part	*Rasa Panchak*
Research work done	1. Saha P, Mandal S, Das A, Das PC, Das S. Evaluation of the anti-carcinogenic activity of *Swertia chirata* Buch. Ham, an Indian medicinal plant, on DMBA-induced mouse skin carcinogenesis model. Phytotherapy Research: An International Journal Devoted to Pharmacological and Toxicological Evaluation of Natural Product Derivatives. 2004 May;18(5):373-8. 2. Barua A, Choudhury P, Mandal S, Panda CK, Saha P. Therapeutic potential of xanthones from *Swertia chirata* in breast cancer cells. Indian Journal of Medical Research. 2020 Mar 1;152(3):285. 3. Saha P, Das S. Highlighting the anti-carcinogenic potential of an ayurvedic medicinal plant, *Swertia Chirata*. Asian Pac J Cancer Prev. 2010 Jan 1;11(6):1445-9. 4. Khan HJ, Ahmad MK, Mahdi AA, Rastogi N, Ansari JA, Shahab U, Khan AR. Evaluation of antiproliferative and antioxidant activity of *Swertia chirata*: implications in breast cancer. International Journal of Research and Development in Pharmacy & Life Sciences. 2016 Jan 15;6(1):2493-501. 5. He QY, Wang R, Sun XC. Cytotoxicity of methanolic extract of *Swertia petiolata* against gastric cancer cell line SNU-5 is *via* induction of apoptosis. South African Journal of Botany. 2017 Mar 1;109:196-202.			
11.	*Ela*	*Elettaria cardamomum* Matom.	Fruit, Fruit seeds	*Rasa -K-M* *Guna -Laghu, Ruksha* *Virya -Sheeta* *Vipaka -Katu* Action on dosha -balances *VataKapha*
Research work done	1. Majdalawieh AF, Carr RI. *In vitro* investigation of the potential immunomodulatory and anticancer activities of black pepper (*Piper nigrum*) and cardamom (*Elettaria cardamomum*). Journal of Medicinal Food. 2010 Apr 1;13(2):371-81. 2. Vutakuri N, Somara S. Natural and herbal medicine for breast cancer using *Elettaria cardamomum* (L.) Maton. IJHM. 2018;6:91-6. 3. Qiblawi S, Al-Hazimi A, Al-Mogbel M, Hossain A, Bagchi D. Chemopreventive effects of cardamom (*Elettaria cardamomum* L.) on chemically induced skin carcinogenesis in Swiss albino mice. Journal of medicinal food. 2012 Jun 1;15(6):576-80. 4. Elguindy NM, Yacout GA, El Azab EF, Maghraby HK. Chemoprotective effect of *Elettaria cardamomum* against chemically induced hepatocellular carcinoma in rats by inhibiting NF-κB, oxidative stress, and ornithine decarboxylase activity. South African journal of botany. 2016 Jul 1; 105:251-8.			
12.	*Gokshur*	*Tribulus terrestris*	Panchang	*Rasa -Madhur* *Guna -Guru, Snigdha* *Virya -Sheeta* *Vipaka -Madhur* Action on dosha - Balances all three *doshas*

(Table 2) cont.....

Sr. No.	Drug	Botanical Name	Useful Part	*Rasa Panchak*
Research work done	1. Angelova S, Gospodinova Z, Krasteva M, Antov G, Lozanov V, Markov T, Bozhanov S, Georgieva E, Mitev V. Antitumor activity of Bulgarian herb *Tribulus terrestris* L. on human breast cancer cells. Journal of BioScience & Biotechnology. 2013 Jan 1;2(1). 2. Wei S, Fukuhara H, Chen G, Kawada C, Kurabayashi A, Furihata M, Inoue K, Shuin T. Terrestrosin D, a steroidal saponin from *Tribulus terrestris* L., inhibits growth and angiogenesis of human prostate cancer *in vitro* and *in vivo*. Pathobiology. 2014;81(3):123-32. 3. Kim HJ, Kim JC, Min JS, Kim MJ, Kim JA, Kor MH, Yoo HS, Ahn JK. Aqueous extract of *Tribulus terrestris* Linn induces cell growth arrest and apoptosis by down-regulating NF-κB signaling in liver cancer cells. Journal of Ethnopharmacology. 2011 Jun 14;136(1):197-203. 4. Sun B, Qu W, Bai Z. The inhibitory effect of saponins from *Tribulus terrestris* on Bcap-37 breast cancer cell line *in vitro*. Zhong yao cai= Zhongyaocai= Journal of Chinese medicinal materials. 2003 Feb;26(2):104. 5. Goranova TE, Bozhanov SS, Lozanov VS, Mitev VI, Kaneva RP, Georgieva EI. Changes in gene expression of CXCR4, CCR7, and BCL2 after treatment of breast cancer cells with saponin extract from Tribulus terrestris. Neoplasma. 2015 Jan 1;62(1):27-33.			
13.	*Guduchi*	*Tinospora cordifolia* Willd. Miers	Stem, Leaves	*Rasa -Kashaya-T Guna -Laghu, Snigdha Virya -Ushna Vipaka -Madhur* Action on dosha - Balance all three *doshas*.
Research work done	1. Diwanay S, Chitre D, Patwardhan B. Immunoprotection by botanical drugs in cancer chemotherapy. Journal of Ethnopharmacology. 2004 Jan 1;90(1):49-55. 2. Tungpradit R, Sinchaikul S, Phutrakul S, Wongkham W, Chen ST. Anticancer compound screening and isolation: *Coscinium fenestratum, Tinospora crispa*, and *Tinospora cordifolia*. Chiang Mai Journal of Science. 2010 Sep 1;37(3):476-88. 3. Maliyakkal N, Udupa N, Pai KS, Rangarajan A. Cytotoxic and apoptotic activities of extracts of *Withania somnifera* and *Tinospora cordifolia* in human breast cancer cells. International Journal of Applied Research in Natural Products. 2013;6(4):1-0. 4. Jayaprakash R, Ramesh V, Sridhar MP, Sasikala C. Antioxidant activity of ethanolic extract of *Tinospora cordifolia* on N-nitrosodiethylamine (diethylnitrosamine) induced liver cancer in male *Wister albino* rats. Journal of Pharmacy & Bioallied Sciences. 2015 Apr;7(Suppl 1): S40. 5. Palmieri A, Scapoli L, Iapichino A, Mercolini L, Mandrone M, Poli F, Giannì AB, Baserga C, Martinelli M. Berberine and *Tinospora cordifolia* exert a potential anticancer effect on colon cancer cells by acting on specific pathways. International journal of immunopathology and pharmacology. 2019 Oct;33:2058738419855567.			
14.	*Gunja*	*Abrus precatorius* Linn.	Root, Leaves, Seeds.	*Rasa -T-Kashay Guna -Laghu,Ruksha Virya -Ushna Vipaka -Katu* Action on dosha - balances *Vata* and *Kapha*

(Table 2) cont.....

Sr. No.	Drug	Botanical Name	Useful Part	*Rasa Panchak*
Research work done				1. Sofi MS, Sateesh MK, Bashir M, Harish G, Lakshmeesha TR, Vedashree S, Vedamurthy AB. Cytotoxic and proapoptotic effects of *Abrus precatorius* L. on human metastatic breast cancer cell line, MDA-MB-231. Cytotechnology. 2013 May 1;65(3):407-17. 2. Sofi MS, Sateesh MK, Bashir M, Ganie MA, Nabi S. Chemopreventive and anti-breast cancer activity of compounds isolated from leaves of *Abrus precatorius* L. 3 Biotech. 2018 Aug 1;8(8):371. 3. Gul MZ, Ahmad F, Kondapi AK, Qureshi IA, Ghazi IA. Antioxidant and antiproliferative activities of *Abrus precatorius* leaf extracts-an *in vitro* study. BMC Complementary and Alternative Medicine. 2013 Dec;13(1):1-2. 4. Lebri M, Tilaoui M, Bahi C, Achibat H, Akhramez S, Fofie YB, Gnahoué G, Lagou SM, Zirihi GN, Coulibaly A, Zyad A. Phytochemical analysis and *in vitro* anticancer effect of aqueous extract of *Abrus precatorius* Linn. Der Pharma Chemica. 2015;7(8):112-7. 5. Bhutia SK, Behera B, Nandini Das D, Mukhopadhyay S, Sinha N, Panda PK, Naik PP, Patra SK, Mandal M, Sarkar S, Menezes ME. Abrus agglutinin is a potent antiproliferative and anti-angiogenic agent in human breast cancer. International Journal of Cancer. 2016 Jul 15;139(2):457-66.
15.	*Haridra*	*Curcuma longa* Linn.	Rhizome	*Rasa - T-K* *Guna - Laghu, Ruksha* *Virya - Ushna* *Vipaka - Katu* Action on dosha – Balances all three *doshas.*
Research work done				1. Buch ZM, Joshi J, Amonkar A, Vaidya AB. Interventional role of Haridra (*Curcuma longa* Linn) in cancer. Clinical cancer investigation journal. 2012 Apr 1;1(2):45. 2. Mohammad P, Nosratollah Z, Mohammad R, Abbas A, Javad R. The inhibitory effect of *Curcuma longa* extract on telomerase activity in A549 lung cancer cell line. African Journal of Biotechnology. 2010;9(6):912-9. 3. Desai AG, Qazi GN, Ganju RK, El-Tamer M, Singh J, Saxena AK, Bedi YS, Taneja SC, Bhat HK. Medicinal plants and cancer chemoprevention. Current drug metabolism. 2008 Sep 1;9(7):581-91. 4. Ye MX, Li Y, Yin H, Zhang J. Curcumin: updated molecular mechanisms and intervention targets in human lung cancer. International journal of molecular sciences. 2012 Mar;13(3):3959-78. 5. Park C, Kim GY, Kim GD, Choi BT, Park YM, Choi YH. Induction of G2/M arrest and inhibition of cyclooxygenase-2 activity by curcumin in human bladder cancer T24 cells. Oncology reports. 2006 May 1;15(5):1225-31.
16.	*Jambu*	*Syzygium cumini* Linn Skeels	Fruits, Seeds, Stem bark, Leaves.	*Rasa -Kashaya-M-A* *Guna -LAghu, Ruksha* *Virya -Sheeta* *Vipaka -Katu* Action on dosha - balances *Kapha* and *pitta*

(Table 2) cont.....

Sr. No.	Drug	Botanical Name	Useful Part	*Rasa Panchak*
Research work done	1. Goyal PK, Verma P, Sharma P, Parmar J, Agarwal A. Evaluation of the anticancer and anti-oxidative potential of *Syzygium cumini* against benzo [a] pyrene (BaP) induced gastric carcinogenesis in mice. Asian Pac J Cancer Prev. 2010 Jan 1;11(3):753-8. 2. Barh D, Viswanathan G. *Syzygium cumini* inhibits growth and induces apoptosis in cervical cancer cell lines: a preliminary study. ecancermedicalscience. 2008;2. 3. Aqil F, Gupta A, Munagala R, Jeyabalan J, Kausar H, Sharma RJ, Singh IP, Gupta RC. Antioxidant and antiproliferative activities of anthocyanin/ellagitannin-enriched extracts from *Syzygium cumini* L.(Jamun, the Indian Blackberry). Nutrition and cancer. 2012 Apr 1;64(3):428-38. 4. Yadav SS, Meshram GA, Shinde D, Patil RC, Manohar SM, Upadhye MV. Antibacterial and anticancer activity of bioactive fraction of *Syzygium cumini* L. seeds. HAYATI Journal of Biosciences. 2011 Sep 1;18(3):118-22. 5. Khodavirdipour A, Zarean R, Safaralizadeh R. Evaluation of the Anti-cancer Effect of *Syzygium cumini* Ethanolic Extract on HT-29 Colorectal Cell Line. Journal of Gastrointestinal Cancer. 2020 Jun 6.			
17.	*Jatiphala*	*Myristica fragrans* Henlt.	Seed, Seed coat, Oil	*Rasa -T-K* *Guna -Laghu,Tikshna* *Virya -Ushna* *Vipaka -Katu* Action on dosha -balances *Kapha&vata*
Research work done	1. Piras A, Rosa A, Marongiu B, Atzeri A, Dessì MA, Falconieri D, Porcedda S. Extraction and separation of volatile and fixed oils from seeds of *Myristica fragrans* by supercritical CO_2: Chemical composition and cytotoxic activity on Caco-2 cancer cells. Journal of food science. 2012 Apr;77(4):C448-53. 2. Prakash E, Gupta DK. Cytotoxic activity of *Myristica fragrans* (Houtt) ethanolic extract against seven human cancer cell lines. Journal of Food and Nutrition Science. 2013;1(1):1-3. 3. Zhang C, Qi X, Shi Y, Sun Y, Li S, Gao X, Yu H. Estimating trace elements in mace (*Myristica fragrans Houtt*) and their effect on uterine cervix cancer induced by methylcholanthrene. Biological trace element research. 2012 Dec 1;149(3):431-4. 4. Kim EY, Choi HJ, Park MJ, Jung YS, Lee SO, Kim KJ, Choi JH, Chung TW, Ha KT. *Myristica fragrans* suppresses tumor growth and metabolism by inhibiting lactate dehydrogenase A. The American journal of Chinese medicine. 2016 Jul 19;44(05):1063-79. 5. Sa-nguanmoo P, Poovorawan Y. *Myristica fragrans* Houtt. Methanolic extract induces apoptosis in a human leukemia cell line through SIRT1 mRNA downregulation. J Med Assoc Thai. 2007;90(11):2422-8.			
18.	*Kanchanar*	*Bauhinia variegate*	Stem Bark, Flowers	*Rasa -Kashaya* *Guna -Laghu, Ruksha* *Virya -Sheeta* *Vipaka -Katu* *Prabhav-Gandamala nashak* Action on dosha – relieve *Kapha* and *Pitta*

(Table 2) cont.....

Sr. No.	Drug	Botanical Name	Useful Part	*Rasa Panchak*
Research work done	1. Rajkapoor B, Jayakar B, Murugesh N, Sakthisekaran D. Chemoprevention and cytotoxic effect of *Bauhinia variegata* against N-nitrosodiethylamine induced liver tumors and human cancer cell lines. Journal of Ethnopharmacology. 2006 Apr 6;104(3):407-9. 2. Mishra A, Sharma AK, Kumar S, Saxena AK, Pandey AK. *Bauhinia variegata* leaf extracts exhibit considerable antibacterial, antioxidant, and anticancer activities. BioMed Research International. 2013 Aug;2013. 3. Rajkapoor B, Jayakar B, Murugesh N. Antitumour activity of *Bauhinia variegata* on Dalton's ascitic lymphoma. Journal of Ethnopharmacology. 2003 Nov 1;89(1):107-9. 4. Agrawal RC, Pandey S. Evaluation of the anti-carcinogenic and antimutagenic potential of *Bauhinia variegata* extract in Swiss albino mice. Asian Pac J Cancer Prev. 2009 Jan 1;10(5):913-6. 5. Rajkapoor B, Jayakar B, Murugesh N. Antitumour activity of *Bauhinia variegata* against Ehrlich ascites carcinoma induced mice. Pharmaceutical biology. 2003 Jan 1;41(8):604-7.			
19.	*Karvellaka*	*Momordica charantia* Linn.	Leaf, Fruit	*Rasa -T-K* *Guna -Laghu, Ruksha* *Virya -Ushna* *Vipaka -Katu* Action on dosha - *Kapha pitta hara*
Research work done	1. Pongnikorn S, Fongmoon D, Kasinrerk W, Limtrakul PN. Effect of bitter melon (*Momordica charantia* Linn) on level and function of natural killer cells in cervical cancer patients with radiotherapy. Journal of the Medical Association of Thailand= Chotmaihet thangphaet. 2003 Jan;86(1):61-8. 2. Raina K, Kumar D, Agarwal R. Promise of bitter melon (*Momordica charantia*) bioactive in cancer prevention and therapy. Seminars in cancer biology 2016 Oct 1 (Vol. 40, pp. 116-129). Academic Press. 3. Weng JR, Bai LY, Chiu CF, Hu JL, Chiu SJ, Wu CY. Cucurbitane triterpenoid from *Momordica charantia* induces apoptosis and autophagy in breast cancer cells, in part, through peroxisome proliferator-activated receptor γ activation. Evidence-Based Complementary and Alternative Medicine. 2013 Oct;2013. 4. Yung MM, Ross FA, Hardie DG, Leung TH, Zhan J, Ngan HY, Chan DW. Bitter melon (Momordica charantia) extract inhibits tumorigenicity and overcomes cisplatin resistance in ovarian cancer cells by targeting the AMPK signaling cascade. Integrative cancer therapies. 2016 Sep;15(3):376-89. 5. Pitchakarn P, Suzuki S, Ogawa K, Pompimon W, Takahashi S, Asamoto M, Limtrakul P, Shirai T. Kuguacin J, a triterpeniod from *Momordica charantia* leaf, modulates the progression of the androgen-independent human prostate cancer cell line, PC3. Food and chemical toxicology. 2012 Mar 1;50(3-4):840-7.			
20.	*Lashuna*	*Allium sativum* Linn.	Bulb, oil	*Rasa - M-L-K-T-K* *Guna - Tikshna, Guru, Snigdha* *Virya - Ushna* *Vipaka - Katu* Action on dosha - *Vata-Kapha shamak*

(Table 2) cont.....

Sr. No.	Drug	Botanical Name	Useful Part	*Rasa Panchak*
Research work done	1. Asemani Y, Zamani N, Bayat M, Amirghofran Z. Allium vegetables for possible future cancer treatment. Phytotherapy Research. 2019 Dec;33(12):3019-39. 2. Li Z, Le W, Cui Z. A novel therapeutic anticancer property of raw garlic extract *via* injection but not ingestion. Cell death discovery. 2018 Nov 21;4(1):1-0. 3. Amagase H, Milner JA. Various garlic sources and their constituents impact 7, 12-dimethylbenz [α] anthracene binding to mammary cell DNA. Carcinogenesis. 1993 Aug 1;14(8):1627-31. 4. Dorant E, van den Brandt PA, Goldbohm RA, Hermus RJ, Sturmans F. Garlic and its significance for human cancer prevention: a critical view. British journal of cancer. 1993 Mar;67(3):424-9. 5. Fleischauer AT, Poole C, Arab L. Garlic consumption and cancer prevention: meta-analyses of colorectal and stomach cancers. The American journal of clinical nutrition. 2000 Oct 1;72(4):1047-52.			
21.	*Lavang*	*Syzygium aromaticum* Linn.	Flower bud	*Rasa -T-K* *Guna-Laghu,snigdha* *Virya -Sheeta* *Vipaka -Katu* Action on dosha – Balance *Pitta&kapha dosha*
Research work done	1. Banerjee S, Panda CK, Das S. Clove (*Syzygium aromaticum* L.), a potential chemopreventive agent for lung cancer. Carcinogenesis. 2006 Aug 1;27(8):1645-54. 2. Dwivedi V, Shrivastava R, Hussain S, Ganguly C, Bharadwaj M. Comparative anticancer potential of clove (*Syzygium aromaticum*)—an Indian spice—against cancer cell lines of various anatomical origin. Asian Pac J Cancer Prev. 2011 Jan 1;12(8):1989-93. 3. Kumar PS, Febriyanti RM, Sofyan FF, Luftimas DE, Abdulah R. Anticancer potential of *Syzygium aromaticum* L. in MCF-7 human breast cancer cell lines. Pharmacognosy research. 2014 Oct;6(4):350. 4. Das A, Harshadha K, Dhinesh Kannan SK, Hari Raj K, Jayaprakash B. Evaluation of the therapeutic potential of a eugenol-a natural derivative of *Syzygium aromaticum* on cervical cancer. Asian Pacific journal of cancer prevention: A.P.J.C.P. 2018;19(7):1977. 5. Ali I, Naqshbandi MF, Husain M. Cell migration and apoptosis in human lung cancer cells by Clove (*Syzygium aromaticum*) dried flower buds extract. Journal of Taibah University for Science. 2019 Dec 11;13(1):1163-74.			
22.	*Methika*	*Trigonella foenum graecum* Linn	Seeds, whole plant	*Rasa -K-T* *Guna -Laghu, Snigdha* *Virya -Ushna* *Vipaka -Katu* Action on dosha - Balances *vata* and *kapha*.

(Table 2) cont.....

Sr. No.	Drug	Botanical Name	Useful Part	*Rasa Panchak*
Research work done				1. Amin A, Alkaabi A, Al-Falasi S, Daoud SA. Chemopreventive activities of *Trigonella foenum* graecum (Fenugreek) against breast cancer. Cell biology international. 2005 Aug;29(8):687-94. 2. Alsemari A, Alkhodairy F, Aldakan A, Al-Mohanna M, Bahoush E, Shinwari Z, Alaiya A. The selective cytotoxic anti-cancer properties and proteomic analysis of *Trigonella Foenum-Graecum*. BMC complementary and alternative medicine. 2014 Dec 1;14(1):114. 3. Hibasami H, Moteki H, Ishikawa K, Katsuzaki H, Imai K, Yoshioka K, Ishii Y, Komiya T. Protodioscin isolated from fenugreek (*Trigonella foenumgraecum* L.) induces cell death and morphological change indicative of apoptosis in leukemic cell line H-60, but not in gastric cancer cell line KATO III. International journal of molecular medicine. 2002 Dec 31;11(1):23-6. 4. El Bairi K, Ouzir M, Agnieszka N, Khalki L. Anticancer potential of *Trigonella foenum* graecum: cellular and molecular targets. Biomedicine & Pharmacotherapy. 2017 Jun 1;90:479-91.
23.	*Neem*	*Azadirachta indica* Ajuss.	Root, bark, Leaves, Fruits, Flowers, Seeds.	*Rasa -T-K* *Guna -Laghu, Ruksha* *Virya -Sheeta* *Vipaka -Katu* Action on dosha - balances *pitta* and *Kapha*
Research work done				1. Mohamed FZ, Basuni MA, Haikel NG. Anti-tumor activity of Neem leaf Extract and Nimbolide on Ehrlich Ascites Carcinoma Cells in Mice. Journal of Molecular Biochemistry. 2019 Jul 28;8(1). 2. Roy MK, Kobori M, Takenaka M, Nakahara K, Shinmoto H, Isobe S, Tsuchida T. Antiproliferative effect on human cancer cell lines after treatment with nimbolide extracted from an edible part of the neem tree (*Azadirachta indica*). Phytotherapy Research. 2007 Mar;21(3):245-50. 3. Roy MK, Kobori M, Takenaka M, Nakahara K, Shinmoto H, Tsuchida T. Inhibition of colon cancer (HT-29) cell proliferation by a triterpenoid isolated from *Azadirachta indica* is accompanied by cell cycle arrest and up-regulation of p21. Planta medica. 2006 Aug;72(10):917-23. 4. Bharati S, Rishi P, Koul A. *Azadirachta indica* exhibits chemopreventive action against hepatic cancer: studies on associated histopathological and ultrastructural changes. Microscopy Research and Technique. 2012 May;75(5):586-95. 5. Othman F, Motalleb G, Peng SL, Rahmat A, Fakurazi S, Pei CP. Extract of *Azadirachta indica* (Neem) leaf induces apoptosis in 4T1 breast cancer BALB/c mice. Cell Journal (Yakhteh). 2011;13(2):107.
24.	*Punarnava*	*Boerhavia diffusa* Linn.	Root, Leaves, Whole plant.	*Rasa - M-T-K* *Guna - Laghu, Ruksha* *Virya- Ushna* *Vipaka - Katu* Action on dosha - Balance all three *dosha*

(Table 2) cont.....

Sr. No.	Drug	Botanical Name	Useful Part	Rasa Panchak
Research work done	1. Srivastava R, Saluja D, Dwarakanath BS, Chopra M. Inhibition of human cervical cancer cell growth by ethanolic extract of *Boerhaavia diffusa* Linn. (punarnava) root. Evidence-Based Complementary and Alternative Medicine. 2011 Jan 1;2011. 2. Sultana S, Asif HM, Nazar HM, Akhtar N, Rehman JU, Rehman RU. Medicinal plants were combating against cancer-a green anticancer approach. Asian Pacific Journal of Cancer Prevention. 2014;15(11):4385-94. 3. Bakrania AK, Nakka S, Variya BC, Shah PV, Patel SS. The anti-tumor potential of herbomineral formulation against breast cancer involves inflammation and oxidative stress. 4. Manu KA, Kuttan G. Anti-metastatic potential of Punarnavine, an alkaloid from *Boerhaavia diffusa* Linn. Immunobiology. 2009 Apr 1;214(4):245-55. 5. Bharali R, Azad MR, Tabassum J. Chemopreventive Action of *Boerhaavia Diffusa* on DMDA-induced Skin Carcinogenesis in Mice. Indian journal of physiology and pharmacology. 2003 Oct 1;47:459-64.			
25.	*Putikaranja*	*Holoptelea integrifolia* Roxb.	Bark	*Rasa -T-K* *Guna -Laghu, Ruksha* *Virya -Ushna* *Vipaka -Katu* Action on dosha - *Kapha-Pitta shamak*
Research work done	1. Guo H, Wang DS, Rizwani GH, Ahmed M, Ahmed M, Hassan A, Xu RH, Mansoor N, Tiwari AK, Chen ZS. Antineoplastic activity of Holoptelea integrifolia (Roxb.) Planch bark extracts (in vitro). Pakistan journal of pharmaceutical sciences. 2013 Nov 1;26(6). 2. Reddy BS, Reddy RK, Naidu VG, Madhusudhana K, Agwane SB, Ramakrishna S, Diwan PV. Evaluation of antimicrobial, antioxidant, and wound-healing potentials of Holoptelea integrifolia. Journal of Ethnopharmacology. 2008 Jan 17;115(2):249-56.3. 3. Kumar V, Singh S, Srivastava B, Bhadouria R, Singh R. Green synthesis of silver nanoparticles using leaf extract of Holoptelea integrifolia and preliminary investigation of its antioxidant, anti-inflammatory, antidiabetic and antibacterial activities. Journal of Environmental Chemical Engineering. 2019 Jun 1;7(3):103094. 4. Dixit P, Pal M, Upreti D. Comparative studies on the analytical and antioxidant activities of the medicinally important stem bark of Holoptelea integrifolia. JPC-Journal of Planar Chromatography-Modern TLC. 2014 Jun 1;27(3):162-5.			
26.	*Saptaparna*	*Alstonia scholaris* R.Br	Stem Bark, Latex, Flowers.	*Rasa -T-K* *Guna -Laghu, Snigdha* *Virya -Ushna* *Vipaka -Katu* Action on dosha - Balances *Kapha&Vata*

(Table 2) cont.....

Sr. No.	Drug	Botanical Name	Useful Part	*Rasa Panchak*
Research work done	1. Baliga MS. Alstonia scholaris Linn R Br in the treatment and prevention of cancer: past, present, and future. Integrative cancer therapies. 2010 Sep;9(3):261-9. 2. Wang CM, Tsai SJ, Jhan YL, Yeh KL, Chou CH. Antiproliferative activity of triterpenoids and sterols isolated from Alstonia scholaris against non-small-cell lung carcinoma cells. Molecules. 2017 Dec;22(12):2119. 3. Surya Surendren P, Jayanthi G, Smitha KR. *In vitro* evaluation of the anticancer effect of methanolic extract of Alstonia scholaris leaves on mammary carcinoma. Journal of Applied Pharmaceutical Science. 2012;2(05):142-9. 4. Sharma V, Mallick SA, Tiku AK. Anticancer activity of Devil tree (Alstonia scholaris Linn.) leaves on Human cancer cell lines. Indian Journal of Agricultural Biochemistry. 2010;23(1):63-5. 5. Jagetia GC, Baliga MS. Evaluation of anticancer activity of the alkaloid fraction of Alstonia scholaris (Sapthaparna) *in vitro* and *in vivo*. Phytotherapy Research: An International Journal Devoted to Pharmacological and Toxicological Evaluation of Natural Product Derivatives. 2006 Feb;20(2):103-9.			
27.	Sharpunkha	*Tephrosia purpurea* Linn. Pers	Root, Whole plant.	Rasa -T-K Guna -Laghu, Ruksha, Tikshna Virya -*Ushna* *Vipak*a -*Katu* Action on dosha - Balances *Vata* and *Kapha*
Research work done	1. Kavitha K, Manoharan S. Anticarcinogenic and anti-lipid peroxidative effects of Tephrosia purpurea (Linn.) In 7, 12-dimethylbenz (a) anthracene (DMBA) induced hamster buccal pouch carcinoma. Indian journal of pharmacology. 2006 May 1;38(3):185. 2. Patel A, Patel A, Patel A, Patel NM. Determination of polyphenols and free radical scavenging activity of Tephrosia purpurea Linn leaves (Leguminosae). Pharmacognosy Research. 2010 May;2(3):152. 3. Hussain T, Siddiqui HH, Fareed S, Vijayakumar M, Rao CV. Chemopreventive evaluation of Tephrosia purpurea against N-nitrosodiethylamine-induced hepatocarcinogenesis in Wistar rats. Journal of Pharmacy and Pharmacology. 2012 Aug;64(8):1195-205. 4. Padmapriya R, Ashwini S, Raveendran R. *In vitro* antioxidant and cytotoxic potential of different parts of Tephrosia purpurea. Research in pharmaceutical sciences. 2017 Feb;12(1):31.			
28.	Shigru	*Moringa oleifera* Linn.	Leaves, Seeds, Fruits, Flowers, Bark.	Rasa -K-T Guna -Laghu,Ruksha,Tikshna Virya -*Ushna* *Vipak*a -*Katu* Action on dosha - Balance *Vata* and Kaha dosha

Sr. No.	Drug	Botanical Name	Useful Part	*Rasa Panchak*
Research work done	1. Hagoel L, Vexler A, Kalich-Philosoph L, Earon G, Ron I, Shtabsky A, Marmor S, Lev-Ari S. Combined effect of Moringa oleifera and ionizing radiation on survival and metastatic activity of pancreatic cancer cells. Integrative cancer therapies. 2019 Mar;18:1534735419828829. 2. Ju J, Gothai S, Hasanpourghadi M, Nasser AA, Ibrahim IA, Shahzad N, Pandurangan AK, Muniandy K, Kumar SS, Arulselvan P. Anticancer potential of Moringa oleifera flower extract in human prostate cancer PC-3 cells *via* induction of apoptosis and downregulation of AKT pathway. Pharmacognosy Magazine. 2018 Oct 1;14(58):477. Baskar AA, Al. Numair KS, Alsaif MA, Ignacimuthu S. *In vitro* antioxidant and antiproliferative potential of medicinal plants used in traditional Indian medicine to treat cancer. redox Report. 2012 Jul 1;17(4):145-56. 3. Waiyaput W, Payungporn S, Issara-Amphorn J, Nattanan T, Panjaworayan T. Inhibitory effects of crude extracts from some edible Thai plants against replication of hepatitis B virus and human liver cancer cells. BMC complementary and alternative medicine. 2012 Dec 1;12(1):246. 4. Yang D, Zhang X, Zhang W, Rengarajan T. Vicenin-2 inhibits Wnt/β-catenin signaling and induces apoptosis in HT-29 human colon cancer cell line. Drug design, development, and therapy. 2018;12:1303.			
29.	Shnoyak	*Oroxylum indicum* Linn.	Root, Bark, Leaves, Stem, Fruits.	Rasa -M-T-K Guna - Laghu Ruksha Virya -*Ushna* *Vipak*a -*Katu* Action on dosha - Balance *Kapha&vata.*
Research work done	1. Kumar DN, George VC, Suresh PK, Kumar RA. Cytotoxicity, apoptosis induction and antimetastatic potential of *Oroxylum indicum* in human breast cancer cells. Asian Pac J Cancer Prev. 2012 Jan 1;13(6):2729-34. 2. Buranrat B, Noiwetch S, Suksar T, Ta-ut A. Inhibition of cell proliferation and migration by Oroxylum indicum extracts on breast cancer cells *via* Rac1 modulation. Journal of Pharmaceutical Analysis. 2020 Feb 12. 3. Zazali KE, Abdullah H, Jamil NI. Methanol extract of Oroxylum indicum leaves induces G1/S cell cycle arrest in HeLa cells *via* the p53-mediated pathway. International Journal of Medicinal Plant Research. 2013;2(7):225-37.			
30.	Tulsi	*Ocimum scantum* Linn.	Leaves, Roots & Seeds	Rasa - K-T Guna -Laghu, Ruksha, Tikshna Virya - *Ushna* *Vipak*a - *Katu* Action on dosha - Balance *Vata* and *Kapha*

(Table 2) cont.....

Sr. No.	Drug	Botanical Name	Useful Part	*Rasa Panchak*
Research work done	1. Manaharan T, Thirugnanasampandan R, Jayakumar R, Kanthimathi MS, Ramya G, Ramnath MG. Purified essential oil from *Ocimum sanctum* Linn. triggers the apoptotic mechanism in human breast cancer cells. Pharmacognosy magazine. 2016 May;12(Suppl 3): S327. 2. Joseph BA, Nair VM. *Ocimum sanctum* Linn. (Holy basil): pharmacology behind its anti-cancerous effect. Int J Pharm Bio Sci. 2013 Apr;4(2):556-75. 3. Bhattacharyya P, Bishayee A. *Ocimum sanctum* Linn. (Tulsi): an ethnomedicinal plant for the prevention and treatment of cancer. Anticancer drugs. 2013 Aug 1;24(7):659-66. 4. Kaushal N, Rao S, Ghanghas P, Abraham S, George T, D'souza S, Mathew JM, Chavali J, Swamy MK, Baliga MS. Usefulness of *Ocimum sanctum* Linn. in Cancer Prevention: An Update. InAnticancer Plants: Properties and Application 2018 (pp. 415-429). Springer, Singapore. 5. Dhandayuthapani S, Azad H, Rathinavelu A. Apoptosis induction by *Ocimum sanctum* extract in LNCaP prostate cancer cells. Journal of medicinal food. 2015 Jul 1;18(7):776-85.			
31.	Yasthimadhu	*Glycyrrhiza glabra* Linn.	Roots	Rasa - Madhura Guna - Guru, Snigdha Virya -Sheeta *Vipak*a - Madhura Action on dosha –*Vata*pittaghna
Research work done	1. Metri K, Bhargav H, Chowdhury P, Koka PS. *Ayurveda* for chemo-radiotherapy induced side effects in cancer patients. Journal of stem cells. 2013 Apr 1;8(2):115. 2. Beriwal VK, Singh B, Thapliyal S, Thapliyal S. A Clinical Evaluation of Guduchi (*Tinospora cordifolia*) and Yashtimadhu (*Glycyrrhiza glabra*) as Chemopreventive Agent in Cancer Treatment. Asian Journal of Oncology. 2019 Jul;5(02):064-71. 3. Pandey S, Verma B, Arya P. A review on constituents, pharmacological activities, and medicinal uses of *Glycyrrhiza glabra*. Pharmaceutical Research. 2017;2(2):26-31. 4. Bahmani M, Rafieian-Kopaei M, Jeloudari M, Eftekhari Z, Delfan B, Zargaran A, Forouzan S. A review of the health effects and uses of drugs of plant licorice (*Glycyrrhiza glabra* L.) in Iran. Asian Pacific Journal of Tropical Disease. 2014;4(S2): S847-9.			

* M- Madhur, A- Amla, L- Lavan, K- *Katu*, T- *Tikta*

A balanced condition of doshas is very important for cancer patients, which can be achieved through *Ayurveda*. Better results are seen when some symptomatic and Rasayana drugs are used. Maintaining a healthy lifestyle is also important during these measures. *Ayurveda* explains specific pathya and apathy for various diseases which should be followed to maintain a healthy lifestyle.

PATHYAPATHYA

1. Add fruit, vegetables, and multi-grain food to the diet.

2. Use Cow's ghee, milk, *etc.*, as much as possible in food.

3. Food enriched with Vitamin D should be used as it exerts a defensive effect in developing tumors.

4. Avoid *Viruddha ahar sevan.*

5. Medicine that stimulates *Agni* (like *sunthi, marich,* or *pippali*) can be used with food to enhance metabolism.

6. Avoid alcohol, tobacco, or other intoxications.

7. One should not overeat.

8. Meditate daily.

9. Create a positive environment and emotions.

10. Exercise daily.

CONCLUSION

Modernization changed lifestyles, including everyday activities. Modern drugs can treat such disorders, but long-term usage might damage key organs. Chemotherapy and radiotherapy are supported worldwide by medicinal herbs. Herbs combined with conventional medicines boost survival, immunological regulation, and quality of life in many clinical studies. Cancer treatments have many negative effects and immunological suppression. This chapter discusses herbs, cancer treatment, and its effects. This chapter briefly discusses cancer-fighting herbs. Here are anticancer research and clinical studies that affected biological pathways. Ayurveda advocates combining medicinal herbs with a diet for better outcomes.

REFERENCES

[1]   Palliyaguru DL, Singh SV, Kensler TW. *Withania somnifera*: From prevention to treatment of cancer. Mol Nutr Food Res 2016; 60(6): 1342-53.

[2]   Shohat B, Gitter S, Abraham A, Lavie D. Antitumor activity of withaferin A (NSC-101088). Cancer Chemother Rep 1967; 51(5): 271.

[3]   Dasgupta A, Kang E, Olsen M, Actor JK, Datta P. Interference of Asian, American, and Indian (Ashwagandha) ginsengs in serum digoxin measurements by a fluorescence polarization immunoassay can be minimized by using a new enzyme-linked chemiluminescent immunosorbent or turbidimetric assay. Arch Pathol Lab Med 2007; 131: 619-21.

[4]   Birla H, Rai SN, Singh SS, *et al. Tinospora cordifolia* suppresses neuroinflammation in parkinsonian mouse model. Neuromolecular Med 2019; 21(1): 42-53.

[5]   Padma VV, Baskaran R, Divya S, Priya LB, Saranya S. Modulatory effect of *Tinospora cordifolia* extract on Cd-induced oxidative stress in Wistar rats. Integr Med Res 2016; 5(1): 48-55.

[6]   Jayakumar T, Hsieh CY, Lee JJ, Sheu JR. Experimental and clinical pharmacology of Andrographis paniculata and its major bioactive phytoconstituent andrographolide. Evid Based Complement Alternat Med 2013; 2013: 846740.

[7]   Rajagopal S, Kumar RA, Deevi DS, Satyanarayana C, Rajagopalan R. Andrographolide, a potential cancer therapeutic agent isolated from Andrographis paniculata. J Exp Ther Oncol 2003; 3(3): 147-58.

[8]   Oda Y. Inhibitory effect of curcumin on SOS functions induced by UV irradiation. Mutation Research Letters 1995; 348(2): 67-73.

[9]   Gururaj AE, Belakavadi M, Venkatesh DA, Marmé D, Salimath BP. Molecular mechanisms of anti-angiogenic effect of curcumin. Biochem Biophys Res Commun 2002; 297(4): 934-42.

[10]   Yoysungnoen P, Wirachwong P, Bhattarakosol P, Niimi H, Patumraj S. Effects of curcumin on tumor angiogenesis and biomarkers, COX-2 and VEGF, in hepatocellular carcinoma cell-implanted nude mice. Clin Hemorheol Microcirc 2006; 34(1-2): 109-15.

[11]   Hao F, Kumar S, Yadav N, Chandra D. Neem components as potential agents for cancer prevention and treatment. Biochimica et Biophysica Acta (BBA)-. Rev Can 2014; 1846(1): 247-57.

[12]   Niture SK, Rao US, Srivenugopal KS. Chemopreventative strategies targeting the MGMT repair protein: augmented expression in human lymphocytes and tumor cells by ethanolic and aqueous extracts of several Indian medicinal plants. Int J Oncol 2006; 29(5): 1269-78.

[13]   Moudi M, Go R, Yien CY, Nazre M. Vinca alkaloids. Int J Prev Med 2013; 4(11): 1231.

[14]   Taher MA, Nyeem MA, Billah MM, Ahammed MM. Vinca alkaloid-the second most used alkaloid for cancer treatment A review. J Physiol Nutr Phys Educ 2017; 2: 723-7.

[15]   Desai SJ, Prickril B, Rasooly A. Mechanisms of phytonutrient modulation of cyclooxygenase-2 (COX-2) and inflammation related to cancer. Nutr Cancer 2018; 70(3): 350-75.

[16]   Kundu JK, Surh YJ. Breaking the relay in deregulated cellular signal transduction as a rationale for chemoprevention with anti-inflammatory phytochemicals. Mutat Res 2005; 591(1-2): 123-46.

[17]   Prashar R, Kumar A, Banerjee S, Rao AR. Chemopreventive action by an extract from *Ocimum sanctum* on mouse skin papillomagenesis and its enhancement of skin glutathione S-transferase activity and acid soluble sulfydryl level. Anticancer Drugs 1994; 5(5): 567-72.

[18]   Baliga MS, Jimmy R, Thilakchand KR, *et al.* *Ocimum sanctum* L (Holy Basil or Tulsi) and its phytochemicals in the prevention and treatment of cancer. Nutrition Cancer 2013; 65(sup1): 26-35.

[19]   Manikandan P, Vinothini G, Priyadarsini RV, Prathiba D, Nagini S. Eugenol inhibits cell proliferation *via* NF-κB suppression in a rat model of gastric carcinogenesis induced by MNNG. Invest New Drugs 2011; 29(1): 110-7.

[20]   Baliga MS, Dsouza JJ. Amla (*Emblica officinalis* Gaertn), a wonder berry in the treatment and prevention of cancer. Eur J Cancer Prev 2011; 20(3): 225-39.

[21]   Nandi P, Talukder G, Sharma A. Dietary chemoprevention of clastogenic effects of 3,4-benzo(a)pyrene by *Emblica officinalis Gaertn.* fruit extract. Br J Cancer 1997; 76(10): 1279-83.

[22]   Dhir H, Roy AK, Sharma A. Talukder G. Modification of clastogenicity of lead and aluminium in mouse bone marrow cells by dietary ingestion of *Phyllanthus emblica* fruit extract. Mutat Res 1990; 241(3): 305-12.

[23]   Sancheti G, Jindal A, Kumari R. Goyal PK. Chemopreventive action of emblica officinalis on skin carcinogenesis in mice. APJCP 2005; 6(2): 197-201.

[24]   Makena PS, Chung KT. Effects of various plant polyphenols on bladder carcinogen benzidine-induced mutagenicity. Food Chem Toxicol 2007; 45(10): 1899-909.

[25]   Zhao T, Sun Q, Marques M, Witcher M. Anticancer properties of Phyllanthus emblica (Indian gooseberry). Oxid Med Cell Longev 2015; 2015:950890.

[26]   Dhongade H, Chandewar AV. Pharmacognostical, phytochemical, pharmacological properties and toxicological assessment of *Phyllanthus amarus*. Int J Biol Adv Res 2013; 4(5): 280-7.

[27]   Lee SH, Jaganath IB, Wang SM, Sekaran SD. Antimetastatic effects of Phyllanthus on human lung

(A549) and breast (MCF-7) cancer cell lines. PLoS One 2011; 6(6): e20994.

[28]   kumar NVR, Joy KL, Kuttan G, Ramsewak RS, Nair MG, Kuttan R. Antitumour and anti-carcinogenic activity of *Phyllanthus Amarus* extract. J Ethnopharmacol 2002; 81(1): 17-22.

[29]   Malvika S, Satyapal S, Lal JM, Mita K. An Ayurveda approach to combat toxicity of chemo-radiotherapy in cancer patients. Int J Res Ayurveda Pharm 2016; 7 (Suppl. 2): 124-9.

[30]   Premalatha B. Sachdanandam P. Regulation of mineral status by *Semecarpus anacardium* Linn. nut milk extract in Aflatoxin B1-induced Hepatocellular Carcinoma. J Clin Biochem Nutr 1998; 25(2): 63-70.

[31]   Pandey R, Maurya R, Singh G, Sathiamoorthy B, Naik S. Immunosuppressive properties of flavonoids isolated from *Boerhaavia diffusa* Linn. Int Immunopharmacol 2005; 5(3): 541-53.

CHAPTER 7

The Classical Ayurveda Anti-Cancer Formulations

Dhirajsingh S. Rajput[1,*]

[1] *Central Council for Research in Ayurvedic Sciences (CCRAS), Ministry of AYUSH, New Delhi, India*

Abstract: Rasoushadhis are special Ayurveda pharmaceutical formulations prepared from metals, minerals, potent herbs, and animal products. These medicines are preferred for severe chronic illnesses which are difficult to cure and life-threatening. Cancer is one such disease that ancient seers of Ayurveda noted. Several Rasoushadhis with potential cytotoxic and cell growth inhibitor actions are recommended for cancer treatment. The present chapter aims to disseminate such formulations, the basis behind their activity, and relevant other formulations that Ayurveda practitioners use to manage Bhaishajya Ratnavali and Rasayogasagar are two important compendia of Ayurveda formulations. Therefore in the present work, the anti-cancer formulations narrated in these two texts are reviewed and compiled. It can be said that the prevalence of cancer in the ancient Indian population was far less, and this may be why the number of anti-cancer formulations is limited. The use of metals and minerals in the form of chelation therapy for cancer can be correlated with Ayurveda anti-cancer Rasoushadhis. Several modern kinds of research on metals, minerals, and herbs contain supportive evidence indicating the rightness of the classical claim of the anti-cancer effect of herbominetal preparation. Relevant information from such research is also presented here. This chapter may be a brief illustrator of the ancient wisdom of anti-cancer formulations.

Keywords: Anti-cancer formulations, Bhaishajya Ratnavali, Herbominetal preparations, Rasoushadhis.

INTRODUCTION

The history of disease is as old as humankind, and so are the efforts for its management. This is why several conditions narrated in ancient traditional healthcare systems are well noted in modern times. Rheumatoid arthritis, tuberculosis, asthma, hemiplegia, diabetes, urinary stones, various skin diseases, and cancer are some diseases the ancient seers of traditional medicine describe. The same are major categories of chronic conditions included in modern medic-

---

* Corresponding author Dhirajsingh S. Rajput: Central Council for Research in Ayurvedic Sciences (CCRAS), Ministry of AYUSH, New Delhi, India; E-mail: dhiraj.ayu@gmail.com

Vaishali Kuchewar, Gaurav Rajendra Sawarkar, Padam Prasad Simkhada & Mahalaqua Nazli Khatib (Eds.)

ine. Cancer is one of the chronic diseases which have been noted cause of mortality in the Global Burden of Diseases by the World Health Organization [1].

The modern system has discovered several advanced technologies to deal with life-threatening diseases such as cancer; however, the unwanted health effects still force science to find a better cure [2]. On the other hand, the traditional system, such as Ayurveda, has dealt with cancer for thousands of years. It is understood that there is a difference between modern medicine and Ayurveda in the way of expressing knowledge and treating disease. For example, cancer has been narrated in Ayurved under the heading *Arbuda* (tumor), *Granthi* (glandular swelling). *Galaganda* (cervical lymphadenopathy) [3]. Therefore, the knowledge of Ayurveda anti-cancer treatment is not as widely known as the recent trend of chemotherapy. To understand the Ayurveda literature for cancer management, it is necessary to know the anti-cancer formulations narrated in Ayurveda and the concept behind the specific combination of ingredients.

In the context of cancer, it can be claimed that the prevalence of this disease was far less during the ancient time because of a healthy lifestyle, healthy diet, far fewer habits of addiction, and no or insignificant use of chemicals in food and cosmetics. Therefore, Ayurveda narrated literature has limited formulations, mostly herbs-mineral preparations. Bhaishajya Ratnavali and Rasayoga Sagar are the two texts of Ayurveda in which the maximum number of formulations from all available classical texts are compiled systematically. Hence in the present chapter, formulations from these two classical texts are taken along with relevant literature and research works.

FORMULATIONS FOR LOCAL APPLICATION

The formulations for local application can be divided into two categories, those which require to be applied with specific media or with particular procedures and the formulations which are like ointment and can be easily used on the site. The location application is preferable in a visible or palpable tumor condition. The generated heat locally and the absorbed phytochemical constituents through the skin may restrict the growth and fasten the decaying mechanism of tumor cells. Time, duration, and thickness for local application of these formulations are to be judged by the physician based on the Arbud and Prakriti patient type. Acharya Govinda Das has compiled 11 formulations for local application in his treatise Bhaishajya Ratnavali. These formulations are depicted in Table **1**.

Table 1. Formulations narrated in Bhaishajya Ratnavali, Galagandadi Rogadhikar for local application in different types of cancer [4].

Sr.	Formulation	Application Media	Indication
1	HinstradiLepa	With Gopitta	Vatagranthi
2	Milk application	Jaloukavacharana and internal administration of Kakolivarga Kashaya	Pittaja Granthi
3	Vikankadi Lepa	*	Kaphaja Granthi
4	Dantimuladi Lepa	*	Kaphaja Granthi
5	Sajjiksharadi Lepa	*	Granthi Arbuda
6	Snigdhamansa Upanah	* (Followed by Nadisweda and Shrunga Raktamokshana)	Vata Arbuda
7	Udumbaradi Lapa	* (followed by Mrudusweda, Upanah, PittaghnaPathya, Virechana)	Pitta Arbuda
8	Mulibhasma and Shankhchurnalepa	*	KaphajArbuda
9	Upodikadi Lepa	*	Kaphaj Arbuda
10	Snuhyadi Lepa	*	All Arbuda
11	Haridradi Lepa	*	Medoarbuda

* Location application media is not required as the formulation is like ointment.

Herbo-Mineral Anti-Cancer Formulations

In Ayurveda pharmaceutics, before the therapeutic utilization of metals and minerals, they are converted into herb-mineral complexes with nanoparticles [5]. Later, these nanoparticles are combined with herbs and utilized for intended purposes. In other words, the nanoparticle or nanomedicines of metal/mineral are the sources of developing desired formulations to treat a disease. Regarding cancer as a primary indication, only two formulations are mentioned in Ayurveda. (Table 2). However, in Rasayogasagar, 17 formulations are noted with a secondary indication as anti-cancer (Fig. 1).

Table 2. Two primary anti-cancer formulations.

S.N	Formulation	Dose	Anupana	References
1	Roudra Rasa	1 Gunja (125 mg)	Honey	Bhaishajya Ratnavali [6]
2	Arbudahara Rasa	1 Gunja (125 mg)	Honey or according to disease complications	Rasachandashu [7]

Formulations	Parada (Mercury)	Gandhaka (Salphur)	Abhraka (Mica)	Swarna Makshika (Chalcopyrite)	Hartala (Orpiment)	Manahshila (Realar)	Swarna (Gold)	Rajata (Silver)	Loha (Iron)	Tamra (Copper)	Tutha (Blue Vitriol)	Naga (Lead)	Shilajatu (Black Bitumen)	Mandura (Rusted Iron)	Vanga (Tin)	Pittala (Brass)	Kaanshya (Bronze)	Kharpar (Calomel)	Kasis (Green Vitriol)	Nagasindoor	(Lead Sulphide)
Amavatari Rasa	+	+	-	-	-	-	-	-	+	+	+	-	-	-	-	-	-	-	-	-	-
Chandra-Prabha Vati(Ii)	-	-	+	-	-	-	-	-	+	-	-	-	-	+	-	-	-	-	-	-	-
Dinardha Rasa	+	+	+	+	+	+	+	+	+	+	+	+	+	+	+	+	+	+	+	+	+
Hemadri Rasa	+	+	+	-	-	-	-	-	-	-	-	-	+	-	-	-	-	-	-	-	-
Kanakagiri Rasa (Ii)	+	+	+	-	-	-	-	+	-	+	-	-	+	-	-	-	-	-	-	-	-
Kamakala Vati	-	-	-	+	-	-	-	-	+	-	-	-	-	+	-	-	-	-	-	-	-
Laxminarayana Rasa (Iii)	+	+	+	-	-	+	+	+	+	-	-	-	+	-	-	+	-	-	-	-	-
Lavanga Paka	+	-	-	-	-	-	-	-	-	+	-	-	-	-	-	-	-	-	-	-	-
Manikya Rasayanama (Ii)	-	-	-	-	-	-	+	+	-	-	-	-	-	-	-	-	-	-	-	-	-
Mohadrivajra Pata Rasa	+	+	+	-	-	-	-	-	-	-	-	+	-	-	-	-	-	-	+	-	-
Nityanada Rasa	+	+	-	-	+	-	-	-	+	+	-	-	-	-	+	-	+	-	-	-	-
Nripatti Vallabha Rasa	+	+	+	-	-	-	-	-	+	+	-	-	-	-	-	-	-	-	-	-	-
Someshwara Rasa (I)	+	+	+	-	-	-	-	-	+	-	-	-	-	-	-	-	-	-	-	-	-
Talkeshwara Rasa (Xv)	-	-	-	-	+	-	-	-	-	-	-	-	-	-	-	-	-	-	-	-	-
Traymbak Abhrakam	-	-	+	-	-	-	-	-	-	-	-	-	-	-	-	-	-	-	-	-	-
Tryushnadi Vati	-	-	+	-	+	-	-	-	+	-	+	-	+	-	-	-	-	-	-	-	-
Yogaottama Vati	-	-	-	+	-	-	-	-	+	-	-	-	+	-	-	-	-	-	-	-	-

Fig. (1). Anti-cancer formulations as per Rasayogasagar.

Basis of Anti-Cancer Combinations

The overall view of all the formulations in Tables **2** and **3** indicates that the formulations are a combination of herbs possessing anti-inflammatory, anti-allergic, anti-hyperlipidemic, rejuvenating, antioxidant, specific organ protective (such as hepatoprotective, nephroprotective, *etc.*), anabolic, *etc.* properties. New drug development found that 48.6% of anti-cancer drugs are derivatives of natural products, *i.e.*, herbs and animal products [8]. Similar natural resources are also utilized in Ayurveda anti-cancer formulations in addition to herbo-mineral nanomedicines, *i.e.*, *Bhasma*. *Bhasma's*are nanomedicines and become a major ingredient in the formulation. Hence these formulations can be divided into metal/mineral-based categories such as *Suvarna Kalpa*(formulations of gold), *Rajata Kalpa* (formulations of silver), *etc.* Understanding the properties of individual metals will help in knowing and rationalizing the basis of Ayurveda anti-cancer hebo-mineral formulation.

Parada Kalpa (Formulations of Mercury)

Here *Parada Kalpa* term indicates *Kupipakwa Rasayana* prepared as per following all classical procedures. In experimental animal research, mercury is used as a cytotoxic agent [9]; however, its cytotoxic action is mild compared to its action on abnormal cancer cells [10]. The studies indicate that *Parada Kalpa* possesses anti-cancer potential but does not show cytotoxic activity against normal cells [11]. In other words, the Ayurveda pharmaceutical procedure may be responsible for nullifying the normal cell cytotoxic potency of mercury, making it more suitable for therapeutic use. Parada is indicated in all types of diseases; hence, with proper combinations, Parada Kalpacan is used in any cancer.

Suvarna Kalpa (Formulations of Gold)

Due to the wide range of therapeutic potentials of Suvarna (gold), it has attracted the modern scientific community's attention for cancer treatment [12]. The significance of *Suvarna* compounds is increasing due to their strong suppressive action overgrowth of tumor cells. Current research claims that gold-based drugs may prove better effective, safe, and therapeutically target-oriented towards specific cancer cells expecting a site-specific delivery mechanism to be created [13]. As mentioned, Ayurvedic formulations contain herbs with specific organ-oriented action. When Suvarna Bhasmais are combined, then in such combination, the particular location-oriented step *Suvarna* is directed.

Rajata Kalpa (Formulations of Silver)

Youngs WJ *et al.* studied the anti-cancer properties of nanoparticle-encapsulated silver carbene and found the antitumor potential in silver carbene [14]. A molecule containing a neutral carbon atom is known as a carbine. The preparative procedure of *Bhasma* involves repeated incineration and trituration in herbal juices. The incineration mechanism converts most of the herbal complex into carbon; the heat and pressure during incineration lead to the formation of the silver-carbon complex. The analytical studies of *RajataBhasma* have established the presence of such complexes [15]. Another study has also found anti-cancer properties of silver in lung cancer cells. In Ayurveda, The affinity of *Rajata* towards the lungs is highlighted by its indication of lung tuberculosis [16]. In general, it can be interpreted that the *Rajata Kalpas* can is specifically used for lung cancer.

Hartal and Manashila Kalpa (Formulations of Arsenic Trisulphide and Bisulphide)

In traditional Indian and Chinese medicine, Arsenic compounds have been used in treating diseases for centuries and recently in malignant tumors [17, 18]. Recent studies have proven that arsenic prohibits cell cycle-related genes in breast cancer cells [19], and inhibits DNA methyltransferase. It restores methylation-silenced genes in human liver cancer cells, thereby helping to treat liver cancer [20] and, through inducing anti-angiogenesis, provides relief in prostate cancer [21]. Modern research indicates that the nanoparticles of *Hartal* and *Manashila* show better cytotoxic effects on cancer cells (especially in skin cancer) compared to simple powder [22, 23]. This observation directs towards using Kupipakwa Kalpa of Hartal and Manashilasuch as Mallasindoor, Samirpannaga Rasa and Talasindoor; for effective preparation of anti-cancer *Hartal* and *Manashila Kalpa.*

Lohaand Mandura Kalpa (Formulations of Iron and Iron Oxide)

Loha and *Mandura Kalpa* have been abundantly used in Ayurveda since the period of Charaka Samhita. The nanoparticle of *Loha* and *Mandura* targets lipid peroxidation [24], increases reactive oxygen species stress [25], and works as a platform to deliver therapeutic siRNA specifically to cancer cells. These attributes not only indicate *Loha* and *Mandura Kalpa* as anti-cancer medicines but also suggest their use as *Yogavahi* to enhance the anti-cancer potential of other metals/minerals. However, *Loha* and *Mandura Kalpa* are health and strength promoters, and the same action is expected to support the cancer patient while continuing the treatment. The prevalence of anemia in cancer patients is around 30% to 90% [26]. Hence treating anemia is also a step in cancer management which implies the significance of *Loha* and *Mandura Kalpa.*

Tamra Kalpa (Formulations of Copper)

Tamra Kalpas are mostly utilized in hepato-biliary diseases [27]. The nanoparticles prepared from copper are found to have cytotoxic potential against lung cancer [28], breast cancer [29], colons, and hepatic cancer [30]. The exact potential of *Tamra Kalpa* in treating cancer is yet to be proven as its utilization frequency is less compared to Gold, Silver, Iron, and Arsenic compounds.

Other Metals/Minerals such as Naga, Vanga, Kasya, Pittal and Shilajatu Kalpa

Naga (Lead), *Vanga* (Tin), and *Shilajatu* (black bitumen) possess rejuvenating and aphrodisiac potential. Rejuvenation action is needed to maintain physical strength as well as to slow down the growth of cancer cells. According to the Ayurved point of view, the aphrodisiac action is indicative of *Shukra Vardhana* (increase in semen quality and quantity), and *Shukra Dhatu* is the source of formation of Oja; which is essential and helpful in combating all kinds of illnesses [31]. *Kasya* (Bronze) and *Pittal* (Brass) formulations are very rare in Ayurveda compendia. The role and utility of these two mixed metals in treating cancer are unknown as there are neither vivid classical claims nor modern research to consider their anti-cancer potential.

WORDS OF PRECAUTION

The pharmaceutical process of Ayurveda herbo-mineral formulations involves several steps such as *Shodhana* (Ayurveda method of metal-mineral and poisonous herb purification), *Jarana* (open pan frying with specific media), *Marana* (incineration to convert into metal/mineral calx) and *Amritikarana* (removing any blemishes left even after all procedures mentioned above). All these processes must be done per classical texts to prepare good quality and safe metal/mineral ingredients for herbo-mineral formulations. Similarly, these formulations should be used with great care regarding dose and dietary regimens. The Rasashastra branch of Ayurveda has described the management of any untoward effect that did not follow the classical guideline [32]. To ensure safety and efficacy, the physician should be aware of these management guidelines. According to Ayurveda, along with internal medication; procedures such as *Virechan* (purgation), *Nasya* (nasal drops), *Swedana* (hot fomentation), *Dhumapan* (medicated herb smoking), *Siravedha* (blood letting), *Agnikarma* (cauterization), *Kshara Prayoga* (use of alkaline, corrosive herb or medicine) and *Lepa* (local application) are to be followed before or during the treatment period [33]. If surgery is required in complicated cancer cases, then the preference should be given to surgery followed by Ayurveda anti-cancer formulations for healing and avoiding reoccurrence. In a nutshell, experience and expertise in using herbo-mineral formulations in managing chronic severe health illnesses such as cancer; are to be taken as a task of utmost causality.

CONCLUSION

Rasoushadhis are Ayurvedic pharmaceuticals manufactured from metals, minerals, potent herbs, and animals. These drugs are preferred for severe chronic conditions that are difficult to treat and potentially lethal. Several Rasoushadhis with cytotoxic and cell growth inhibitor capabilities are recommended for cancer treatment. This chapter shares such formulations, their mechanisms, and additional Ayurvedic disease-management formulas. Ayurvedic formulation compendia include Bhaishajya Ratnavali and Rasayogasagar. Ayurvedic anti-cancer Rasoushadhis are linked to chelation therapy metals and minerals. Metal, mineral, and plant studies with relevant study result support herbominetal preparation's anti-cancer activity.

REFERENCES

[1]   World Health Organization. The global burden of disease 2004. Available from: https://www.who.int/healthinfo/global_burden_disease/GBD_report_2004update_part2.pdf?ua=1

[2]   Peppercorn J. Financial toxicity and societal costs of cancer care: distinct problems require distinct solutions. Oncologist 2017; 22(2): 123-5.

[3]   Nidansthan ATSHV, Ed. Sushruta Sushruta Samhita (Purvardha) Shastri A. 9th ed. Varanasi: Chaukhamba Sanskrit Sansthan 1995; p. 270.

[4]   Das G. Bhaishajya Ratnavali. Shastri H, Ed. Galagandadi Rogadhikar. Reprint ed. Delhi. Motilal Banarasidas Publication 1983; pp. 541-2.

[5]   Pal D, Sahu CK, Haldar A. Bhasma: the ancient Indian nanomedicine. J Adv Pharm Technol Res 2014; 5(1): 4-12.

[6]   Dash MK, Joshi N, Dubey VS, Dwivedi KN, Gautam DNS. Screening of anti-cancerous potential of classical Raudra rasa and modified Raudra rasa modified with hiraka bhasma (nanodiamond) through FTIR & LC-MS analysis. J Comp Integrative Med, 2022; 19(3): 669–682. [http://dx.doi.org/10.1515/jcim-2021-0410]

[7]   Ruhila A, Yadav P, Ruknuddin G, Prajapati PK. Review of anti-cancer activity of metals and minerals. J Ayu Med Sci 2018; 3(3): 405-12. [http://dx.doi.org/10.5530/jams.2018.3.20]

[8]   Newman DJ, Cragg GM. Natural products as sources of new drugs over the 30 years from 1981 to 2010. J Nat Prod 2012; 75(3): 311-35.

[9]   Hossain KF, Rahman MM, Sikder MT, Hosokawa T, Saito T, Kurasaki M. Selenium modulates inorganic mercury induced cytotoxicity and intrinsic apoptosis in PC12 cells. Ecotoxicol Environ Saf 2021; 207: 111262.

[10] Kannan N, Shanmuga SS, Balaji S, Amuthan A, Anil NV, Balasubramanian N. Physiochemical characterization and cytotoxicity evaluation of mercury-based formulation for the development of anti-cancer therapeuticals. PLoS One 2018; 13(4): 1-13.

[11] Nafiujjaman M, Nurunnabi M, Saha SK, Jahan R, Lee YK, Rahmatullah M. Anticancer activity of Arkeshwara Rasa-A herbo-metallic preparation. Ayu 2015; 36(3): 346-50.

[12] Gabbiani C, Casini A, Messori L. Gold (III) compounds as anti-cancer drugs. Gold Bull 2007; 40(1): 73-81.

[13] Nardon C, Boscutti G, Fregona D. Beyond platinums: gold complexes as anti-cancer agents. Anticancer Res 2014; 34(1): 487-92.

[14] Youngs WJ, Knapp AR, Wagers PO, Tessier CA. Nanoparticle encapsulated silver carbene complexes and their antimicrobial and anti-cancer properties: a perspective. Dalton Trans 2012; 41(2): 327-36.

[15] Bhavani MD, Raju M, Sridurga C, Subbaiah KV. Analytical standardization of Rajata Bhasma. Int J Res AYUSH and Pharmace Sci 2018; 1: 229-38.

[16] Vagbhata, Rasaratnasamuchchaya. Tripathi I, Ed. 3rd ed., Varanasi: Choukhamba Sanskrit Sansthan; 2009, pp. 418.

[17] Zheng L, Jiang H, Zhang ZW, et al. Arsenic trioxide inhibits viability and induces apoptosis through reactivating the Wnt inhibitor secreted frizzled related protein-1 in prostate cancer cells. OncoTargets Ther 2016; 9: 885-94.

[18] Ji H, Li Y, Jiang F, et al. Inhibition of transforming growth factor beta/SMAD signal by MiR-155 is

involved in arsenic trioxide-induced anti-angiogenesis in prostate cancer. Cancer Sci 2014; 105(12): 1541-9.

[19] Moghaddaskho F, Eyvani H, Ghadami M, *et al.* Demethylation and alterations in the expression level of the cell cycle–related genes as possible mechanisms in arsenic trioxide–induced cell cycle arrest in human breast cancer cells. Tumour Biol 2017; 39(2): 1-16.

[20] Cui X, Wakai T, Shirai Y, Yokoyama N, Hatakeyama K, Hirano S. Arsenic trioxide inhibits DNA methyltransferase and restores methylation-silenced genes in human liver cancer cells. Hum Pathol 2006; 37(3): 298-311.

[21] Javed Z, Khan K, Rasheed A, *et al.* MicroRNAs and Natural Compounds Mediated Regulation of TGF Signaling in Prostate Cancer. Front Pharmacol 2021; 11: 613464.

[22] Lin M, Wang Z, Zhang D. Preparation of orpiment nanoparticles and their cytotoxic effect on cultured leukemia K562 cells. J Nanosci Nanotechnol 2007; 7(2): 490-6.

[23] Wu J, Shao Y, Liu J, Chen G, Ho PC. The medicinal use of realgar (As4S4) and its recent development as an anti-cancer agent. J Ethnopharmacol 2011; 135(3): 595-602.

[24] Jaganjac M, Sunjic SB, Zarkovic N. Utilizing iron for targeted lipid peroxidation as anti-cancer option of integrative biomedicine: A short review of nanosystems containing iron. J Antioxidants 2020; 9(3): 191.

[25] Huang G, Chen H, Dong Y, *et al.* Superparamagnetic iron oxide nanoparticles: amplifying ROS stress to improve anti-cancer drug efficacy. J Theranostics 2013; 3(2): 116-26.

[26] Knight K, Wade S, Balducci L. Prevalence and outcomes of anemia in cancer: a systematic review of the literature. Am J Med 2004; 116(7): 11-26.

[27] Panda AK, Bhuyan GC, Rao MM. Ayurvedic intervention for hepatobiliary disorders: current scenario and future prospect. J Tradit Med Clin Natur 2017; 6(1): 1-5.

[28] Sankar R, Maheswari R, Karthik S, Shivashangari KS, Ravikumar V. Anticancer activity of *Ficus religiosa* engineered copper oxide nanoparticles. Mater Sci Eng C 2014; 44(1): 234-9.

[29] Sivaraj R, Rahman PK, Rajiv P, Narendhran S, Venckatesh R. Biosynthesis and characterization of *Acalypha indica* mediated copper oxide nanoparticles and evaluation of its antimicrobial and anti-cancer activity. Spectrochim Acta A Mol Biomol Spectrosc 2014; 129: 255-8.

[30] Hassanien R, Husein DZ, Al-Hakkani MF. Biosynthesis of copper nanoparticles using aqueous Tilia extract: antimicrobial and anti-cancer activities. Heliyon 2018; 4(12): e01077.

[31] Rani I, Satpal P, Gaur MB. Physiological evaluation of oja in relation to bala: A critical review. Int J Basic Appl Res 2018; 8(10): 276-83.

[32] Kavyashree BP, Sharma VS. A critical analysis of Bhasmasevana doshas and it's management. World J Pharm Pharm Sci 2017; 6(2): 348-91.

[33] Das G. Bhaishajya Ratnavali. Shastri H. Ed. Galagandadi Rogadhikar. Reprint ed. Delhi. Motilal Banarasidas Publication 1983; pp. 542.

CHAPTER 8

Application of Dincharya, Rutucharya and Yoga for the Prevention and Management of Cancer

Sadhana Misar Wajpeyi[1,*]

[1] *Department of Kayachikitsa, Mahatma Gandhi Ayurved College Hospital and Research Centre, Salod(H), Wardha, Maharashtra, India*

Abstract: Cancer is a group of diseases having an uncontrolled unregulated division of abnormal cells that tend to spread to all other parts of the body. It is observed that about 80-90 percent of the causes of cancer include unhealthy diet, behavioral habits, and environmental factors that can be prevented. Cancer is not described in Ayurveda, but in Brihatatrayi, there is a description of Granthi and Arbuda, which can be correlated with cancer due to the similarity in nature and clinical course. In Ayurveda, there are three major causes of any ailment: Kala Parinam, Pragyaparadha, and AsatmendriyarthaSamyoga. All of this can be prevented by adopting a healthy lifestyle. Hence there is a need to focus on a healthy lifestyle to manage and prevent cancer. Concept of Primordial prevention: The holistic approaches of Swasthavritta like Healthy dietary and behavioral habits, Dincharya, Ritucharya, not restraining non-suppressible urges and holding suppressible desires, Good conduct, Yoga, Pranayama, Meditation, and Shatkarma purifying procedures, all come under primordial prevention. This is the prevention of the risk factors by optimizing lifestyles associated with cancer by following the holistic principles of Ayurveda. Various research studies also proved that these principles of Ayurveda are helpful in the prevention and recovery of cancer patients. On the basis of the conclusion from the literature and available research on cancer, it can be said that adopting the holistic principles of Ayurveda is beneficial in preventing the risk of various types of cancers.

Keywords: Arbud, Ahar, Cancer, Diet, Dincharya, Exercise, Granthi, Meditation, Nidra, Pranayama, Ritucharya, Stress, Yoga.

INTRODUCTION

There is an intimate association between an individual's lifestyle and the state of health and disease. Lifestyle is a way of living that is a routine activity of an individual, which mainly involves dietary (*Aahar*) and behavioral (*Vihara*) that is both physical as well as mental practices. According to W.H.O. (1948), "Health is

---

[*] **Corresponding author Sadhana Misar Wajpeyi:** Department of Kayachikitsa, Mahatma Gandhi Ayurved College Hospital and Research Centre, Salod(H), Wardha, Maharashtra, India; E-mail: sadhanamisar@gmail.com

Vaishali Kuchewar, Gaurav Rajendra Sawarkar, Padam Prasad Simkhada & Mahalaqua Nazli Khatib (Eds.)

a state of complete physical, mental, and social well-being and not merely an absence of disease or infirmity" [1]. *Acharya Sushruta* stated that *"Swastha* (Health) means an individual having balance and normal activities of the *Tridoshas, Agni* (digestive power), seven *Dhatu* (body tissues), *Malas* (excretory products) with having calm *Atma* (Soul), *Mana* (Mind) and *Indriya* (sense organs).

Cancer is a cluster of ailments having an uncontrolled unregulated division of abnormal cells that tend to spread in all other parts of the body. An unhealthy lifestyle, environmental factors, family history, and genetics are risk factors for the occurrence of cancers. Free radicals, natural byproducts of metabolism, are responsible for oxidative stress, which damage the normal cellular structure and function. The continuous process of generating these natural byproducts in the body is going on, and the factors mentioned above accelerate their production. The antioxidant defense system in the body protects the body if these are within normal physiological levels [2]. This antioxidant defense system of the body can be increased by following Ayurveda's holistic principles, which help prevent cancer. Worldwide, cancer is the second most important cause of death. In old times, cancer was believed to be originating from unknown reasons. Still, nowadays, due to progress in medical science, it is observed that about 80-90 percent of the causes of cancer include unhealthy diet, behavioral habits, and environmental factors that can be prevented [3]. Cancer is not described in Ayurveda, but in *Brihatatrayi*, there is a description of *Granthi* and *Arbuda,* which can be correlated with cancer due to the similarity in nature and clinical course. In Ayurveda, there are three major causes of any ailment: *Kala Parinam, Pragyaparadha*, and *Asatmendriyartha Samyoga. Kala Parinama* refers to the *Samyaka* and *Asamyaka Yoga* of different seasons. All of this can be prevented by adopting a healthy lifestyle. Hence, there is a need to focus on a healthy lifestyle to manage and prevent cancer. In Ayurveda, lifestyle is described in the form of *Dinacharya, Ritucharya,* and *Sadvritta*. These are designed based on balancing functions of '*Doshas*', *Dhatu*, '*Agni'*, and '*Mala'*. Acharya Charak described the three *Upasthambhas* (supporting pillars), *Aahar* (Food), *Nidra* (Sleep), and *Brahmacharya* (Celibacy) for the maintenance of good health [4].

THE PREVENTIVE MEASURES FOR CANCER

The Role of Aahar (Diet) in Preventing Cancer

Aahar is considered important among all three *Upasthambhas;* hence it has been given the first place. Inappropriate and unhealthy dietary practices lead to the majority of diseases. If an individual had not taken food properly, it will lead to *Mandagni,* which is a root cause of all diseases. Acharya Charaka described that the quantity of food depends on the strength of *Agni* (digestive fire), *Ritu* (Seasonal changes), and *Vaya* (age) of a person. *Viruddha Aahar* (Incompatibility of food) is a unique concept described by Acharya Charaka. According to this, *Aahardravyas* become incompatible due to their mutually contradictory qualities of 18 types [5]. One should avoid consuming incompatible food, which is one of the major dietary factors responsible for cancer pathogenesis.

Acharya Charak described *Ashta Aahar Vidhi Viseshayatana* that is the eight aspects of Dietetics, the factors responsible for the wholesome and unwholesome effect of the *Aahar*, and methods of *Aaharsevana* (rule for the intake of diet) that should be considered before taking food [6]. Thus food taken in proper quantity by following all laws and regulations stated in Ayurveda will help balance dosha, dhatu, and mala, thereby keeping us healthy, which is important in preventing cancer-like diseases.

Acharya Charaka described Aahar *Vidhi Vidhana*, the general principles of taking *Aahar*, and stated that all should follow these rules while consuming the food to remain healthy and enhance the span of life. For maintaining the equilibrium of *Doshas,* consumption of all six *Rasas* in proper quantity is essential. Excess or less consumption of particular *Rasa Aahar* leads to aggravation and vitiation of *Doshas*. As per Ayurveda, the imbalance of doshas is one of the major causes of the pathogenesis of cancer-like diseases. Therefore, *Shadras Aahar* is considered the best. Improper dietary habits lead to the formation of free radicals in the body, which cause damage to DNA and other parts of human cells leading to a risk of cancer. *Pathyapathya* is another concept described in Ayurveda. *Pathya* (wholesome) *Aahar* that is *Hitkar* and *Apathya* (unwholesome) *Aahar* that is *Ahitakar* should also be considered while taking food. In case of cancer, high caloric fat diet, red meat, canned food, beverages, refined sugar, and excess salt should be avoided. Food rich in plant sources like fruits and vegetables high fiber diet should be consumed [7].

Globally it is estimated that 20-60% of cancers are mainly caused due to dietary factors, and around one-third of mortality is due to cancer in Western countries. The World Health Organization stated that avoiding risk factors and implementing proven preventive measures can help reduce the occurrence of cancer by up to 30-50%. As per the 2012 American Cancer Society (ACS) Guidelines, among these evidence-based measures, there is a close relation between healthy dietary habits and a reduction in deaths due to cancer. Numerous observational studies recommended that an unhealthy diet is an important risk factor for cancer. Evidence from these researches indicated that increased fruit, vegetable, and grain consumption reduces the risk of cancer. Various research studies have recognized the above 500 dietary components as possible modifiers of cancer. Intake of vitamins, minerals and antioxidant-rich food like green vegetables and fruits reduces cancer risk [8]. From research studies, it was recommended that for the prevention of cancer, energy-dense foods rich in fat contents, carbohydrate diets like bakery products, chocolates, polished cereals, sugar-rich food, processed food, red meat, canned food with additives like preservatives, coloring and flavoring agents, beverages and alcohol should be avoided. Eating plant-origin items like fruits, vegetables, and whole grains with a limiting high-fat diet should be taken.

Similarly, high salt intake, processed meats, and moldy cereals or pulses should be avoided. Obesity is a modifiable risk factor for many non-communicable diseases like cancer. Essential and non-essential-allelochemicals of plant foods and zoochemical of animal foods may be physiologically significant modifiers. Various research-based evidence proved the importance of balanced healthy food and adequate exercise in cancer prevention. It is also stated that unhealthy dietary habits, a sedentary lifestyle, excessive intake of alcohol, and smoking increase the risk of cancer [9].

A research study on nutritional factors proposed to reduce the risk of prostate cancer concluded that compounds like carotenoids, dithiolthiones, flavonoids, glucosinolates, isothiocyanates, allyl sulfhydryls, and fermentable fibers have been found to control experimentally induced cancer. Vegetables and fruits rich in vitamins, minerals, and phytochemicals (*e.g.*, carotenoids, flavonoids, phytoestrogens, and isothiocyanates) proved to have anti-carcinogenic properties by retarding the development of cancer cells, inhibiting tumor promotion, reducing oxidative damage of DNA by antioxidant properties [10].

The Role of *Vihar* (Behavioral) in Preventing Cancer

Vihar, a behavioral regimen, includes *Dinacharya, Ritucharya, Sadvritta, Nidra, Brahmacharya, Achar Rasayana, Yoga*, and *Pranayam* practices.

In Ayurveda, *Dincharya* (daily regimen) is described as one of the health-promotive and preventive measures for diseases [11]. It helps maintain a state of equilibrium of three Doshas, Dhatu, Mala, and the Agni along with Atma, Mana, and Indriya, which helps maintain positive health. As per Ayurveda imbalance of the Doshas, Dhatu, Mala, and Agni is the cause of the pathogenesis of all diseases like cancer.

Dinacharya and its Applicability

Bramhamuhurta Uttishte

Bramhamuhurta, i.e., 96 min before sunrise, is the ideal time to wake up in the morning after completing the night's sleep. Scientifically before sunrise, the air is fresh with minimum pollution and high oxygen saturation; that is *Pranvayu*. This helps in easy and fast oxygen absorption in the blood, which nourishes body tissues rapidly. This helps in increasing antioxidants and helps in reducing oxidative stress, thereby reducing the risk of cancer. In the early morning, serotonin is released, which calms the mind, enhances concentration, and increases the feeling of well-being and happiness. Stress is a major factor in the etiology of cancer. Serotonin has a role in both innate as well as adaptive immunity. It stimulates the monocytes and lymphocytes and thus influences the secretion of cytokines. Low doses of serotonin can inhibit tumor growth via the decrease of blood supply to the tumor [12].

Ushnajalapana

Ushna jalapana proved to lukewarm water that helps in *Vatanulomana* (causes normal *gati* to *Vata*), removes constipation, and enhances digestive fire.

Malotsarjana

As per Ayurveda, in the morning, Vata dosha is dominant; hence this is a proper time to eliminate feces and urine. These are *Adharniya vegas* that help clean the body by removing waste from the body. It helps in enhancing digestive power and prevents constipation. A research study stated that patients with chronic constipation had elevated risks of colorectal and other GI cancers, and non-GI cancers were moderately increased only in the short term, especially for ovarian cancer [13, 14].

Nasya (Therapeutic Nasal Oil Pulling Therapy)

Instilling Oil or *Ghrita* in the nostrils helps remove all accumulated *Doshas* from *Shirpradesh*. *Pratimarsha Nasya* with *Anutaila* or *Katutaila* is advised for daily *Nasya* practice. It prevents the entry of dust particles into the nasal tract. It directly stimulates the olfactory nerve endings and improves nerves' function.

Abhyanga (Oil Massage)

Massage with oil is very beneficial to the whole of the body and scalp every day. It nourishes whole body by improving blood circulation, and helps eliminate metabolic wastes from the body. It softens the body by reducing dryness and removing stiffness of the joints. It also strengthens the muscles, ligaments, and joints.

Shirobhyanga (Massage to *Shirpradesha*) calms the mind by relieving stress and anxiety. It enhances memory and concentration. *Padabhyanga* (Massage to feet) removes dryness, roughness, stiffness, and tiredness. It helps in inducing sound sleep. *Karnapurana* (Instilling oil in the ear) helps prevent pain, stiffness, and various ear disorders.

These daily practices of Nasya and abhyanga help promote health by improving blood circulation and functions of all body organs. Abhyanga has been found helpful in reducing anxiety, stress, and depression [15]. The effect has been drawn in a clinical study on cancer patients. It helps in detoxification and relaxation. It helps reduce anxiety and mental stress by calming the mind and inducing good sleep. This help in reducing the risk of cancer as stress is one of the major causes of it [16].

Exercise And Chankramana

Regular exercise increases strength, helps clear all strotas (channels) of the body, and improves blood circulation. This improves the efficiency of vital organs, increases digestive fire, and helps remove excessive fat. Obesity is one of the major causes of cancer, so exercise helps to remove it. Many research studies stated an inverse relationship between physical activity and cancer occurrence. Epidemiologic data from 73 kinds of research carried out worldwide point toward a 25% decrease in the risk of breast cancer amongst most women doing physical exercise compared to those who are not exercising. A meta-analysis of 19 research studies documents the inverse relationship between kidney cancer and physical activity. Similarly, many research studies established the protective role of exercise in reducing the risk of many other cancers, like pulmonary, uterine, colon, and prostate cancer. Daily regular exercise causes certain changes in the body, like reduction in the inflammatory response, improvement in the immune mechanism, and increase in natural antioxidants; these all help reduce the risk of cancer [17, 18].

Ritucharya (Seasonal Regimen)

The human body being an integral unit of nature, the seasonal changes affect human physiology too. *Ritucharya* is one of the ways to deal with these changes and to help in keeping good health. The atmospheric conditions influence changes in *Dosha, Bala*, and *Agni*. Due to changes in the external environment, the *Tridosha* passes through three phases, *i.e., Sanchaya, Prakopa,* and *Prashama,* as shown in Table **1**. If the regimen of *Ritucharya* is followed properly, aggravated *Doshas* get pacified.

Table 1. Stages of *Doshas* as per *Ritu*.

Dosha	Sanchay (Accumulation)	Prakopa (Aggravation)	Prashama (Pacification)	Elimination Procedure
Vata	Grishma	Varsha	Sharad	Basti
Pitta	Varsha	Sharad	Hemant	Virechana
Kapha	Shishir	Vasant	Grishma	Vaman

So one must follow the dietary and behavioral regimen described in *Ritucharya* to maintain the equilibrium of *Dosha, Dhatu, Agni,* and *Bala*. The imbalance of dosha is a major cause of diseases like cancer. The purification processes indicated in particular ritu help in detoxification by removing carcinogenic substances and also aid in reducing oxidative stress, a major cause of cancer. In *Samhita,* indications, and contraindications of food and behavior are stated, which should be followed to prevent diseases caused due to seasonal changes. One of the etiological factors of cancer involves environmental factors like environmental pollutants and radiation. Radiation is mainly associated with skin cancer, so adopting a seasonal regimen will help reduce cancer risk [19].

Nidra (Sleep)

Sleep is one of the three *Upastambhas* essential for good health. Acharya Charak described that happiness, suffering, nutrition, health, wasting, weakness, intelligence, ignorance, life, and death all depend on proper and adequate sleep. But excessive sleep takes away the happiness and longevity of human beings. Melatonin is involved in circadian regulation and facilitation of sleep, inhibiting cancer development and growth and enhancing immune function. Melatonin is mainly secreted during the night and can reduce oxidative stress, which is the major factor for cancer. It affects the immune system by enhancing both natural and acquired immunity; thus, it can prevent cancer. Sleep disturbances can lead to immune suppression and a shift to the predominance of cancer-stimulatory cytokines. Some studies suggest that a shortened nocturnal sleep duration is associated with a higher risk of breast cancer development [20].

Brahmacharya-Curbing and Controlling Desires

Besides *Aahar* and *Nidra, Brahmacharya* is the third component of *Trayopstambha*. *Brahmacharya* is the avoidance of sexual acts physically, mentally, and verbally under any circumstances. Celibacy is one of the best enhancers of longevity. It promotes nourishment, pleasantness, and happiness. *Shukra Dhatu* is preserved in the body, so the strength of the body is increased. Rules and regulations described in Ayurveda for the regulated sexual activity should be followed to maintain good health.

Rasayana (Rejuvenation Therapy) and *Sadvritta* (Rules of Good Conduct)

Rasayana is a rejuvenation therapy described in Ayurveda that helps in the maintenance as well as promotion of health. *Rasayana* provides nutrition at all levels. Various types of Rasayana therapy deal not only with drug therapy but also include a specific nutritional diet and good behavioral conduct. *Ajasrika Rasayana* mainly deals with using nutritious diets like *Ghrita* and milk. They help strengthen bodily tissues with immune modulators and antioxidant properties, which help reduce cancer risk. *Achar Rasayana* includes practicing good behavioral conduct. The code of *Achara Rasayana* keeps the aspirant free from emotional disturbances and allows a less stressful life leading to health and happiness. Reducing stress helps prevent cancer, as stress is a major factor associated with cancer. Cancer is caused by an abnormal growth of body cells. The major reason for the abnormal growth of body cells is reduced strength and immunity. Exercise helps one to increase the body's strength as well as immunity power. Hence it is advised that exercise should be done regularly by everybody.

Roganutpadakabhavas (Preventive Aspects of Diseases)

In *Roganutpadaka bhavas,* Acharya Charaka described *Adharaniya* and *Dharaniyavega,* which is responsible for causing diseases. *Vegadharan* means the suppression of natural urges. Natural urges are of two types, *Dharniya* (suppressible) and *Adharniya* (non-suppressible). There are 13 non-suppressible urges like *Mutra* (urination), *Mala* (defecation), *Shukra* (semen), *Vata* (flatus), *Chhardi* (vomiting), *Shwayathu* (sneezing), *Udgar* (eructation), Jrumbha (yawning), *Kshudha* (hunger), *Truta* (thirst), *Aashru* (tears) and *Nidra* (sleep). According to Ayurveda, *Vega-vidharan* is a major cause of various ailments. Suppression of non-suppressible urges can lead to multiple systemic disorders. *Manasika Vegas*-like *Lobha* (Greediness), *Shoka* (Sorrow), *Bhaya* (Fear), *Krodha* (Fury), *Ahankara* (Ego), *Nirlajjata* (Shamelessness), and Irshya (Envy) are suppressible *Vegas*. These *Manasika Vegas* affect mental as well as physical health. Mind and body influence each other. The mind urges must be suppressed to maintain sound mental health, thereby reducing stress, the major factor for cancer [21].

Role of Yoga- (Asana, Pranayam, and Meditation)

Yoga is an 8-fold (*Ashtanga Yoga*) path to control the mind. It includes *Yama* (moral doctrines), *Niyamas* (disciplines), *Asanas* (postures), *Pranayama* (regulated controlled breathing), *pratyahara* (withdrawal of the senses), *Dharana* (concentration), *Dhyana* (meditation), and *Samadhi* (transcendence) [22].

Asana, Pranayama, and Dhyana practices are mainly useful for preventing lifestyle disorders. The *Asanas,* a particular posture, helps to improve flexibility and strength of the body, whereas *Pranayama* facilitates controlled breathing and easy movement of *Pranavayu* into the body. *Dhyana,* that is meditation relaxes and calms the mind, thus giving a feeling of well-being [23, 24].

The evidence collected through yoga research revealed the health benefits of *Yoga* on different aspects of the physical, mental, and spiritual health, supporting its use in promoting the health. Regular various research conducted showed significant improvement in physiological parameters of the body after *Yoga* like a reduction in the resting heart rate, systolic and diastolic blood pressure, increase in Force Vital Capacity, Forced Expiratory Volume in the first second (FEV1), Peak Expiratory Flow Rate, reduction in Body Mass Index, Reduction in Fasting Blood Sugar, total serum cholesterol, serum triglycerides, serum low-density lipoprotein levels, and the significant increase in High-Density Lipoprotein. It showed activation of the hypothalamic-pituitary-adrenal axis and decrease in self-reported stress, anxiety, fatigue, depression as well as increase in mindfulness, rise in Plasma levels of Brain-Derived Neurotrophic Factors, and increase in the level of the cortisol awakening response. It also showed psychologically beneficial effects like Parasympathetic activity, which superseded sympathetic activity and improved mental health and cognitive benefits [25]. Numerous Yoga studies have shown reduction in cortisol, inflammatory cytokines, and improved natural killer cell counts. It showed improvement in the quality of life; thus, these studies proved that practicing *Yoga* daily helps prevent lifestyle-related disorders, mainly cancer. In some researches, it was demonstrated that *Pranayama* induces relaxation, and increases antioxidant defense and NK cell in the body, thus may have a preventive role against cancer. It was also suggested that *Pranayama* might delay cancer progression and improve survival and quality of life [26, 27].

Dhyana

Dhyana, that is, meditation, is the most important part of *Yoga* practice. This technique includes specific postures, attention, and concentration by avoiding distraction. It helps to calm the mind thus maintaining the psychological balance. It helps in enhancing overall health and well-being. It removes negative thoughts from the mind and is endowed with positive ones. Research studies proved that meditation is the only activity that reduces blood lactate, a marker of stress and anxiety. The calming hormones melatonin and serotonin are increased by meditation, and the stress hormone cortisol is decreased. It helps to relieve anxiety and stress, the major causes of lifestyle disorders, mainly cancer. This helps in preventing cancer. Poor sleep quality has been associated with various lifestyle disorders. Research proved that regular yoga practice significantly affects anxiety, depression, chronic pain, and stress - all common contributors to sleep problems. Further studies showed that daily *Yoga* could help promote better sleep [28].

Shatakarma (Six Yogic Purification Techniques)

Shatakarma is a term described in *Hatha Yoga Pradipika* in which six yogic purification techniques like *Dhauti, Basti, Neti, Nauli, Trataka,* and *Kapal Bhati* are described. These internal cleansing techniques help to keep the body clean, strong, and healthy. They help remove toxins from the body, thus prevents blocking the flow of prana in the body. Practicing *Shatkarma* internally purifies the body, which makes *Pranayama* and meditation practice easy and more beneficial. Detoxification helps remove byproducts of metabolism having carcinogenic properties from the body and helps prevent cancer.

CONCEPT OF PRIMORDIAL PREVENTION

The holistic approaches of Swasthavritta like Healthy dietary and behavioral habits, *Dincharya, Ritucharya*, not restraining non-suppressible urges and holding suppressible desires, Good conduct, *Yoga, Pranayama*, Meditation, and *Shatkarma* purifying procedures, all come under primordial prevention. Primordial prevention is a novel concept that is the prevention of the development of risk factors in the first place with lifestyle only. It means to prevent the occurrence of the risk factors by optimizing lifestyles associated with cancer by following the holistic principles of Ayurveda.

It helps in boosting immunity. The immune system usually protects the body from the harmful effects of pathogens or abnormal cells, including cancer cells. Cancer cells arise daily, typically due to a genetic predisposition or environmental influences but are usually eliminated by the immune system.

Research studies advocated that many cell types belonging to the innate (NK cells and macrophages) and the adaptive (T and B cells) immune systems seem to be involved in cancer control. Lymphocytes, including T cells, T regulatory (T reg) cells, natural killer (NK) cells, and their cytokine release patterns are implicated in both primary prevention and secondary prevention of breast cancer [29].

CONCLUSION

Cancer is a group of diseases characterized by uncontrolled cell division that can infiltrate all body parts. Diet, behavior, and environmental factors can prevent cancers. Cancer is not mentioned in Ayurveda, although Brihatatrayi describes Granthi and Arbuda, which are similar to cancer. Ayurveda attributes any sickness to Kala Parinam, Pragyaparadha, and Asatmendriyartha Samyoga. Healthy living prevents this. Cancer care and prevention must prioritize a healthy lifestyle. Preventive principle includes healthy nutrition and behavior, Dincharya, Ritucharya, refraining from non-suppressible needs and holding suppressible desires, good conduct, yoga, pranayama, meditation, and shatkarma purification rites. Avoiding cancer-linked lifestyles and following Ayurvedic holistic principles prevent risk factors. Numerous studies have shown that these Ayurvedic principles can prevent cancer and also help in recovery of cancer patients. Ayurvedic holistic principles can reduce the risk of several cancers, according to cancer literature and studies.

REFERENCES

[1]   Park's Textbook of Preventive and Social Medicine, edited by K.Park, Chapter 2, published by M/s Banarsidas Bhanot, edition 2013.

[2]   Corthay A. Does the immune system naturally protect against cancer? Front Immunol 2014; 5: 197. [http://dx.doi.org/10.3389/fimmu.2014.00197]

[3]   Bray F, Ferlay J, Soerjomataram I, Siegel RL, Torre LA, Jemal A. Global cancer statistics 2018: GLOBOCAN estimates of incidence and mortality worldwide for 36 cancers in 185 countries. CA Cancer J Clin 2018; 68(6): 394-424.

[4]   Navya S, Shetty RK. Nagesh KA. A Review on the concept of Trayopastambha with special reference to Brahmacharya. Journal of Ayurveda and Integrated Medical Sciences 2020; 5(04): 341-6.

[5]   Zambare SV. Viruddha ahara the unique concept of ayurveda. Int J Ayurveda Pharma Res 2017; 5(3).

[6]   Chaudhari DP, Kinage PR. Importance of aahar-vidhi-visheshayatana for prevention of life style disorders: a review. World J Pharm Res 2018; 7(13): 235-49.

[7]   Neeraj AK, Prasad UN. A review article on karka roga (cancer) in terms of agadatantra. Int Ayurvedic Med J 2017. Available from: http://www.iamj.in/posts/images/upload/2046_2052.pdf

[8]   Key TJ, Schatzkin A, Willett WC, Allen NE, Spencer EA, Travis RC. Diet, nutrition, and the prevention of cancer. Public Health Nutr 2004; 7(1a): 187-200.

[9]   Pal D, Banerjee S, Ghosh AK. Dietary-induced cancer prevention: An expanding research arena of emerging diet related to healthcare system. J Adv Pharm Technol Res 2012; 3(1): 16.

[10]   Chan JM, Gann PH, Giovannucci EL. Role of diet in prostate cancer development and progression. J Clin Oncol 2005; 23(32): 8152-60.

[11]   Chaudhary M, Rana JK. Role of dincharya regimen towards attaining positive health. International Journal of Ayurvedic and Herbal Medicine 2017; 7(5): 2923-7.

[12]   Karmakar S, Lal G. Role of serotonin receptor signaling in cancer cells and anti-tumor immunity. Theranostics 2021; 11(11): 5296.

[13]   Power AM, Talley NJ, Ford AC. Association between constipation and colorectal cancer: systematic review and meta-analysis of observational studies. Official journal of the American College of

Gastroenterology| ACG 2013; 108(6): 894-903.

[14]   Sundbøll J, Thygesen SK, Veres K, *et al.* Risk of cancer in patients with constipation. Clin Epidemiol 2019; 11: 299.

[15]   Falkensteiner M, Mantovan F, Müller I, Them C. The use of massage therapy for reducing pain, anxiety, and depression in oncological palliative care patients: a narrative review of the literature. International Scholarly Research Notices 2011.

[16]   Klaunig JE. Oxidative stress and cancer. Curr Pharm Des 2018; 24(40): 4771-8.

[17]   Lemanne D, Cassileth B, Gubili J. The role of physical activity in cancer prevention, treatment, recovery, and survivorship. Oncology (Williston Park) 2013; 27(6): 580-5.

[18]   Davies NJ, Batehup L, Thomas R. The role of diet and physical activity in breast, colorectal, and prostate cancer survivorship: a review of the literature. Br J Cancer 2011; 105(1): S52-73.

[19]   Thakkar J, Chaudhari S, Sarkar PK. Ritucharya: Answer to lifestyle disorders. Ayu 2011; 32(4): 466.

[20]   Blask DE. Melatonin, sleep disturbance and cancer risk. Sleep Med Rev 2009; 13(4): 257-64.

[21]   Purushotham A, Bains S, Lewison G, Szmukler G, Sullivan R. Cancer and mentalhealth—a clinical and research unmet need. Ann Oncol 2013; 24(9): 2274-8.

[22]   Saraswati SM, Saraswati SS. Hatha Yoga Pradipika. Yoga Publications Trust 1998.

[23]   Akhtar P, Yardi S, Akhtar M. Effects of Yoga on functional capacity and well being. Int J Yoga 2013; 6(1): 76.

[24]   Sharma RA, Gupta N, Bijlani RL. Effect of yoga-based lifestyle intervention on subjective well-being. Indian J Physiol Pharmacol 2008; 52(2): 123-31.

[25]   Nambinarayanan T, Thakur S, Krishnamurthy N, Chandrabose A. Effect of yoga training on reaction time, respiratory endurance, and muscle strength. Indian J Physiol Pharmacol 1992; 36(4): 229-33.

[26]   Bower JE, Woolery A, Sternlieb B, Garet D. Yoga for Cancer patients & survivors. Cancer Contr 2005; 12(3): 165-71.

[27]   Nagendra HR. Cancer: Prevention and rehabilitation through Yoga. Int J Yoga 2018; 11(1): 1.

[28]   Thordardottir K, Gudmundsdottir R, Zoëga H, Valdimarsdottir UA, Gudmundsdottir B. Effects of yoga practice on stress-related symptoms in the aftermath of an earthquake: a community-based controlled trial. Complement Ther Med 2014; 22(2): 226-34.

[29]   Standish LJ, Sweet ES, Novack J, *et al.* Breast cancer and the immune system. J Soc Integr Oncol 2008; 6(4): 158-68.

CHAPTER 9

Applied Aspect of Dooshivisha in the Perspective of Cancer

Sonali Chalakh[1,*]

[1] Department of Agadtantra, Mahatma Gandhi Ayurved College Hospital & Research Center, Wardha, Maharashtra, India

Abstract: Agadtantra is a specialized Ayurveda branch that deals with toxicity management. This specialized branch has given the novel concept of Dooshivisha. It is a transformable state of *Visha* (poison) which any type of poison can attain if it is not eliminated from the body completely. Today every individual is frequently exposed to many toxic substances, mostly carcinogenic. Polycyclic hydrocarbons, nitrosamine, pyrogenic compounds and many others are now known to be potent mutagens and carcinogens. These carcinogens enter the body through air, water, radiation, drugs, cosmetics and reflect deposit in the body as a Dooshivisha and slowly vitiate all the Dosha & saptadhatu (seven Dhatu). After studying the etiological factor of cancer in the context of Ayurveda and modern medicine, it is seen that most of the etiological factors and pathology of cancer come under these headings. Radiotherapy and chemotherapy are the only lines of treatment for cancer, but they produce harmful toxic effects along with their beneficial effects. Management of cancer is made easy by adopting a therapeutic approach of Dooshivisha. Various Agadkalpas are useful to reduce or vanish latent toxicity. The integrated system of modern medicine with Dooshivisha management means the application of Agada will be helpful for prevention, minimizing the side effects of conventional therapies, and improving the quality of life of cancer patients.

Keywords: Agad, Cancer, Dooshivisha, Visha.

INTRODUCTION

CONCEPT OF *DOOSHIVISHA*

In Ayurveda, three sources of poisoning are explained in the context of Agadtantra. It is categorized as Sthavar (vegetative), Jangam (animate), and Krutrim (artificial poison). Along with this, ancient seers mentioned a novel concept of poisoning, *i.e.,* Dooshivisha, which means the transformable stage of any poison. It is defined as poison from any source, if not fully eliminated from

---

* **Corresponding author Sonali Chalakh:** Department of Agadtantra, Mahatma Gandhi Ayurved College Hospital & Research Center, Wardha, Maharashtra, India

Vaishali Kuchewar, Gaurav Rajendra Sawarkar, Padam Prasad Simkhada & Mahalaqua Nazli Khatib (Eds.)

the body, gets transformed into another form and retains in the body for a longer period [1]. This poison does not produce any immediate symptoms as Kapha Dosha envelops it due to its low potency. It lays dormant condition and gets spread slowly all over the body. After absorption, it vitiates *Dosha* and then vitiates *saptadhatu* (cells/tissue). In the concept of *Dooshivisha,* the normal functioning of Dhatu gets disturbed (cellular change), and physiological changes are seen in terms of signs and symptoms in a particular system or organ (Table **1**).

Table 1. Causes of cancer concerning Visha (poison).

Source as per Ayurveda	As per Modern
SthavarVisha	Algae, Moulds (*Aspergillus Flavus* & *Aspergillus parasiticus*) - Aflatoxine
	Pteridiumaquilinum - Ptaquiloside
Artificial poison	**Insecticides-**Organophosphate, Carbamate, DDT, **Fungicides – Pentachlorophenol, Creosote** Rodenticides, Herbicides
	Industrial chemical – Hydrocarbons, Alcohol, Aldehydes, Metals, Aromatic amines, Nitro compounds

PATHOPHYSIOLOGY OF CANCER

Due to industrialization and modernization, people are exposed to a large amount of many harmful chemicals every day. Environmental exposure is one of the most significant causes of cancer; as per the WHO and IARC (international agency of cancer research) report, it is estimated that 7-19% of cancer are due to exposure to toxic substances. In the late 1700s, a link between cancer and chemical was found by English surgeon PercivallPott. He observed that chimney soot contains polycyclic aromatic hydrocarbons, and many chimney sweeps suffer from scrotum cancer by exposure to soot [2].

A wide range of physical, chemical, and biological agents have been associated with increased cancer risk. As per the toxicological point of view, all these agents come under the artificial poison category. Common examples are coal tar products, arsenic, radon, asbestos, formaldehyde, and benzene. The body gets exposed to these agents by the air that we breathe, the food that we eat, the water that we drink, and our lifestyle choices. After exposure to the carcinogenic agents, they may be absorbed and distributed all over the body, retained in the transformable stage, or converted into inert form and excreted from the body. The agent that gets absorbed possesses the ability to interact with our genomes in multiple ways and can affect cancer initiation, progression, and aggression. This means these agents can induce genetic and epigenetic alterations in the host tissue.

Hence the process of carcinogenesis evolved over a while. The time from the first cell change to the time the cancer is detected is called a latency period.

CLASSIFICATION OF CARCINOGEN [3]

Based on the mechanism, a carcinogen is of two types: one is genotoxic, and the second is epigenetic. Genotoxic is direct-acting which alters the genes through the interaction with DNA. Epigenetics does not act directly on genetic materials. Genotoxic is further classified into three groups, Direct or primary carcinogen-chemicals now work without any bioactivation; Procarcinogen –chemicals that, after biotransformation, become carcinogenic; Inorganic carcinogenic. Epigenetics is also categorized into subgroups; Co-Carcinogen –these chemicals increase the effectiveness of carcinogen when they are administered together; Promoter- it will not induce cancer itself but increase the response of carcinogen when applied after it; Solid-state –works by an unknown mechanism but physical form vital to effect, Hormone- it alters the endocrine balance and acts as a promoter, or Immunosuppressors (Fig. **1**).

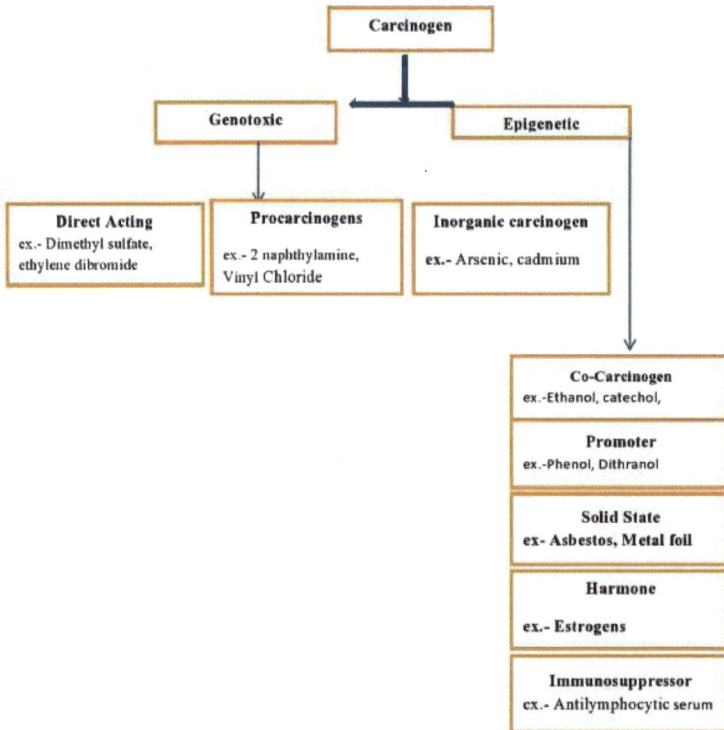

Fig. (1). Classification of carcinogen.

CORRELATION OF CANCER IN THE PERSPECTIVE OF DOOSHIVISHA

Dooshivisha is retained in the body in the latent stage, and when a favorable condition (weakened immunity) develops, it produces various symptoms. Manifestation varied from Jwara to the development of Arbud. When it is retained in Amashaya (stomach), it produces diseases due to the derangement of Vata – Kapha and when it is in Pakwashay (colon), it produces diseases of deranged Vata- Pitta [4]. Hence Dooshivisha is a broad concept under which cumulative toxicity, chronic toxicity, carcinogenicity, and free radicles are all grouped together (Table **2**).

Table 2. Symptoms developed due to Dooshivisha when it is present in Rasadi Dhatu: [5].

Sr No.	Dhatu	Symptoms
1	Rasa	Aruchi, Ajirna
2	Rakta	Kushtha, Visarpa,(all types of skin diseases)
3	Mansa	Arbud
4	Meda	Granthi
5	Asthi	AdhidantyadiVikar
6	Majja	Tamodarshan
7	Shukra	-

As per conventional science, the stages of poisoning are acute and chronic. Acute poisoning occurs when exposure to the poison is on one occasion or during a short period. Chronic poisoning is a long-term repeated or continuous exposure to a toxin in which symptoms do not occur immediately or after every exposure, the patient gradually becomes ill after a long latent period. Chronic poisoning most commonly occurs in the poisons that bio-accumulate or are biomagnified such as metals like mercury, cadmium, and pesticides.

HOW TOXIC SUBSTANCES/CHEMICALS AFFECT THE BODY

The chemicals causing the cancer are known as chemical carcinogens. These chemicals are found in everyday items like cosmetics, daily care products, food preservatives, and pesticides. A few well-known chemicals causing cancer are aromatic hydrocarbons like benzene, aromatic amines, and some inorganic and organic compounds like lead and nickel.

These chemicals enter body tissue through inhalation, ingestion, and skin absorption. Cancer does not produce in every person exposed to these chemicals.

Still, it depends on several factors, including the types of chemicals, their duration and amount of exposure, and individual genetic background. The absorption of these chemicals can take place by active or passive transport and also depends on the physicochemical properties of the substance. The substance absorbed by the lungs is first circulated all over the body by blood and then reaches the liver in the later stage; those absorbed orally pass through the liver and are then distributed in the body (Table **3** and **4**). After absorption, some chemicals directly act on DNA, but most of them undergo the process of metabolism. Through an enzymatic process, some convert into an inert form, and some act as procarcinogens (Fig. **2**). These chemicals disturb the body's normal functioning by disturbing protein structurally and enzymatically, damaging DNA, and reacting in the cell with oxygen to form free radicals, which damage DNA [6].

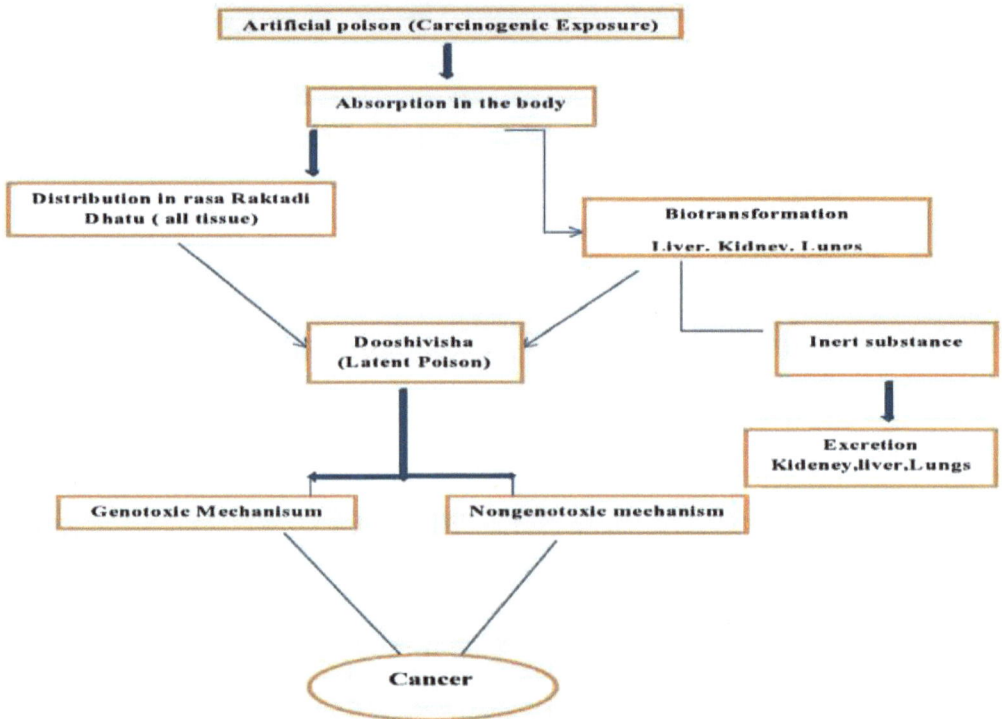

Fig. (2). Artificial poisoning.

Table 3. Chemical carcinogen and its mechanism of action [7].

Group	Compound	Mechanism of Action
Metals	Arsenic, Cadmium, Nickel	Oxidative stress It inhibits DNA repair pathways and nucleotides excision repair, Histone acetylation and DNA hypermethylation.

(Table 3) cont.....

Group	Compound	Mechanism of Action
Polycyclic aromatic compound	Benzopyrene	Form adduct with purine bases of DNA, mainly resulting in transversion.
Aromatic amines	2- napthyamine,4-aminobiphenyls	The genotoxic compound increases the rate of cell duplication.
Halogenated compounds	Trichloroethylene	Somatic mutation, modification of cell cycle pathways.
N-nitroso compounds	N- Nitrsodimethylamine	Forms adducts at N- and O- atoms in the D.N.A. base.
Carbamates	N- methylcarbamate esters	Chromosome aberration, gene mutation, cell transformation.
Natural carcinogen	Aflatoxin B1, Asbestos	Form adducts with guanine, react with R.N.A. and protein
Anticancer drugs	Alkylating agents	Interstrand and intrastandcross link

People in close contact with these chemicals are more prone to produce cancer because of their occupations.

Table 4. Occupational exposure to toxic substances causing cancer.

Sr No.	Carcinogen	Occupational Uses/Sources	Types of Cancer
1	Asbestos	Found in Construction, Roofing Papers, Friction Lining, Floor Tile, Fire Resistant Textile	The gastrointestinal tract, Lungs, Larynx
2	Arsenic	• Component of Fungicides, Algaecides, Medication, Alloys, Electrical and Semiconductor Device • A byproduct of metal Smelting Animal dips, electrical and semiconductor device	Lung, Skin, Haemangiosarcoma, Liver
3	Cadmium	Metal Painting and Coating, Batteries, found in solders	Prostate
	Nickel	Ferrous Alloys, Stainless–Steel Welding Byproduct, Nickel Plating, Ceramics, Batteries	Lung, Nose
4	Exhaust Gas From Engine	IC Engine Exhaust Gas	Lung, Bladder
5	Benzene	Printing, Paint, Rubber, Industry, Dry Cleaning, Adhesive, Coating, Detergent, lithography	Leukemia, Hodgkins Lymphoma
6	Beryllium And Its Compound	Nuclear Reactor, Aerospace Application, Lightweight Alloys, Missile Fuel	Lung

(Table 4) cont.....

Sr No.	Carcinogen	Occupational Uses/Sources	Types of Cancer
7	Hexavalent Chromium Compound	Paints, Pigments, Preservatives	Lung
8	Radon And Its Decay Product	Quarries and Mines Uranium Decaycellars and Poorly Ventilated Places	Lung
9	Ethylene Oxide	Rocket Propellant, Fumigant for Food Stuff And Textiles, Ripening Agents for Fruits And Nuts, Sterilant for Hospital Equipment.	Leukemia
10	Vinyl Chloride	Adhesive for Plastic, Refrigerant, Production For Polyvinyl Chloride	Liver, Haemangiosarcoma
11	Tobacco Smoke, Passive Smoking	-	Lung

PREVENTION OF CANCER WITH DOOSHIVISHA MANAGEMENT [8]

Ayurveda emphasizes the preventive as well as therapeutic aspects for the eradication of morbid tissue, protection of healthy cells from toxicity, and promotion of regeneration of healthy tissue. Depending on the level of medical care, Anticancer treatment has five-categories: preventive, prophylactic, curative, palliative, and supportive. Cancer is a latent phase of poison/chemicals; hence manipulation of carcinogenic substances could be made easy by adopting a therapeutic approach of Dooshivisha. In the context of *Dooshivisha* management, Detoxification is the first line of principle that includes *Vaman* (emesis)/Virechan purificatory procedures, which remove the toxin deposited in the body as in cancer, toxin clearance mechanism gets compromised. After purification, natural compounds that prevent cancer have special characteristics like strengthening the immune system, boosting the detoxification mechanism and fighting the free radicals that cause mutational changes are essential for extending the body. In Agadtantra, various Agadkalpas are mentioned, which are useful to reduce or vanish toxicity (Table **5**).

Table 5. Formulation used for the management of Dooshivisha.

Sr. No.	Formulation
1	Ajitagad
2	PanchgavyaGhrut
3	PatoladiGhrut
4	BilwadiGutika
5	DooshivishariGutika

Sr. No.	Formulation
6	DashangGutika
7	DevamrutGutika

In conventional science, radiotherapy and chemotherapy are effective lines of treatment for cancer management but, at the same time, produce harmful toxic effects. The integrated approach of modern medicine with Dooshivisha management means the application of Agada will be helpful to minimize the side effects of conventional therapies and improve the quality of life.

The formulation mentioned under the context of Dooshivisha has hepatoprotective, nephroprotective, radioprotective, and antioxidant properties, which are needed for managing cancer. One of the most commonly used formulations for Dooshivisha mangment is Dooshivishari Agad. For cancer management, the formulation needed has the property of strengthening the immune system, preventing the spread of cancerous cells, creating an unfavorable environment for cancer growth, means high oxygen levels, detoxifying the body, and fighting free radicles that cause mutational changes. After reviewing the pharmacological activity of Dooshivishari Agad, it is found that it fulfills all the criteria needed for managing cancer (Table **6**).

Hence, applying an integrated approach of Ayurveda and conventional medicine helps prevent and fight cancer.

Table 6. Pharmacological activity of ingredients of Dooshivishari Agad.

Sr no.	Drug Name	Botanical Name	Pharmacological Action in Terms of Cancer
1	Pimpali	Piper longum	Immunomodulatory Hepatoprotective Anticancer activity Anti-oxidative, anti-apoptotic, and restorative ability against cell proliferative mutagenic response
2	Dhyamaka	Cymbopogon martini.	Antioxidant
3	Jatamansi	Nardostachysjatamansi	Hepatoprotective Activity Antioxidant Activity Antiestrogenic activity
4	Ela	Elattaria Cardamum	Anticancer Activity AntioxidentActivity
5	Lodhra	Symplocosracemosa	Anticancer activity Antioxidant Activity Hepato-protective activity

(Table 6) cont.....

Sr no.	Drug Name	Botanical Name	Pharmacological Action in Terms of Cancer
6	Katunatam/shyonak	Oroxylum indicum	Hepato-protective activity Anticancer activity Immuno-stimulating activity Gastro-protective
7	Tagar	Valerianawallichii	Radio-protective activity Anti-oxident Cytotoxic activity
8	Kuth	Saussurea lappa.	Anticancer activity Immuno-modulatory activity Hepato-protective Angiogenesis activity
9	Mulethi	Glycyrrhiza glabraLinn.	Antioxidant Hepato-protective Anticancer Activity Immunomodulator
10	Chandan	Pterocarpus santalinusLinn.f.	Hepatoprotective Antioxident Anticancer Activity
11	Suvarchika	Potassium nitrate	-
12	Gairik	Red ochre	-

CONCLUSION

Air, water, radiation, pharmaceuticals, cosmetics, and food products include carcinogens that deposit as Dooshivisha and eventually vitiate all Dosha and Saptadhatu (seven Dhatu). Most cancer etiology and pathology fall within Ayurveda and modern medicine, according to research. Radiotherapy and chemotherapy are the sole cancer treatments. However, they have pros and cons. Dooshivisha therapy streamlines cancer treatment. Agadkalpas diminish latent toxicity. Agada can prevent cancer, reduce the side effects of conventional therapy, and improve cancer patients' quality of life.

REFERENCES

[1]   Murthy K.S. Shastri, Choukhamba Sanskrit Sasnthana Varanasi, Kalpsthana. Sushrut, Sushrut Samhita, Chapter 2, 2007; 33: 42.

[2]   Gatto NM. Environmental carcinogens and cancer risk. Cancers. 2021; 13(4):622.

[3]   Munjal Y. API textbook of medicine vol 2, Association of a physician of India, ninth ed 2012, pp 1561.

[4]   Deepa P, Nataraj HR, Anushree CG, Akshatha KS. A critical review on Dooshivishari Agada: A herbo mineral formulation. Int J Ayurveda Pharma Res 2022; 10(10): 70-77.
       [http://dx.doi.org/10.47070/ijapr.v10i10.2576]

[5]   Shastri A, Ed. editor, Sushruta Samhita, Kalpsthana, 2/29, Varanasi, Choukhamba Sanskrit Sasnthana, Reprint 2007, 424.

[6]   Gerald NW, Stephen SH, James SF, Allan HC, Lawrence AL. Environmental and chemical carcinogenesis. Semin Cancer Biol 2004; 14(6): 473-86.

[7]   Oliveira PA, Colaço A, Chaves R, *et al.* Chemical carcinogenesis. An Acad Bras Cienc 2007; 79: 593-616.

[8]   Chalakh S. Cancer in perspective of dooshivisha (latent poisoning) w.s.r. to possible role of dooshivishari agada in treating cancer. IJAPC 2018; 9(2): 383-94.

SUBJECT INDEX

A

Acid 13, 26, 36, 41, 43
　acetic 36
　bile 41
　chebulagic 43
　ellagic 43
　gallic 43
　uric 13
Action 41, 42, 45, 65, 70
　anti-proliferation 42
　aphrodisiac 70
　cell growth inhibitor 65
　chain-breaking antioxidant 41
　mitogenetic 45
　radioprotective 45
Activities 22, 41, 44, 45, 46, 81
　antimetastatic 44
　chemoprotective 44, 45, 46
　effective radioprotective 45
　immunostimulant 44
　immunostimulatory 41
　neurological 22
　regulated sexual 81
Adjuvant chemotherapy 12
Anemia 12, 42, 70
Angiogenesis inhibitors 5, 9, 14, 15
Angiopoietin 41
Antidiuretic hormone 42
Antioxidant 41, 43, 44, 45, 68, 79, 93
　activity 43
　effects 45
　natural 79
Antiproliferative activities 44
Apoptosis 5, 6, 40, 41, 43, 45
　activities 45
Ayurveda 39, 66, 71
　anti-cancer treatment 66
　herbo-mineral formulations 71
　herbs 39
Ayurvedic disease-management formulas 71

B

Bethesda system 34
Bhasma'sare nanomedicines 68
Blood 7, 28, 79
　cancer 7, 28
　circulation 79
Bowel mucosa 10
Brain-derived neurotrophic factors 82
Breast cancer 11, 13, 20, 33, 42, 70, 79, 83
　cells 20, 70
　Screening 33
　tumors 42
Brush biopsy 31, 33, 36

C

Calming hormones melatonin 83
Camellia sinensis 20
Cancer 3, 5, 8, 10, 11, 13, 25, 33, 34, 36, 37, 43, 45, 70, 76, 78, 79, 87
　abdominal 10
　bladder 11
　bone 10
　cervical 8, 33, 34, 45
　gastric 43
　hepatic 70
　kidney 79
　lip 3
　metastasis 3
　oral 33, 36, 37, 43
　ovarian 78
　pathogenesis 25, 76
　scrotum 87
　solid tumor 5, 8
　therapy 13
Carbohydrate diets 77
Carcinogenesis 13, 43, 88
Carcinogenic 41, 87
　agents 87
　effects 41
Carcinomas 3, 5, 7, 15, 36, 41

www.ingramcontent.com/pod-product-compliance
Lightning Source LLC
Chambersburg PA
CBHW041720210326
41598CB00007B/714